MW00619408

Introduction to Healthcare Management

Sharon B. Buchbinder, RN, PhD
and
Nancy H. Shanks, PhD

Charles R. McConnell, MBA, CM

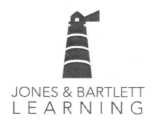

JONES & BARTLETT
LEARNING

World Headquarters
Jones & Bartlett Learning
40 Tall Pine Drive
Sudbury, MA 01776
978-443-5000
info@jblearning.com
www.jblearning.com

Jones & Bartlett Learning Canada
6339 Ormindale Way
Mississauga, ON L5V 1J2
Canada

Jones & Bartlett Learning
International
Barb House, Barb Mews
London W6 7PA
United Kingdom

Jones & Bartlett Learning books and products are available through most bookstores and online booksellers. To contact Jones & Bartlett Learning directly, call 800-832-0034, fax 978-443-8000, or visit our Web site at www.jblearning.com.

Substantial discounts on bulk quantities of Jones & Bartlett Learning publications are available to corporations, professional associations, and other qualified organizations. For details and specific discount information, contact the special sales department at Jones & Bartlett Learning via the above contact information or send an email to specialsales@jblearning.com.

All persons and entities in situations depicted are fictitious and any resemblance to any person living or dead or to any actual entity or situation is purely coincidental.

Copyright © 2012 by Jones & Bartlett Learning, LLC

All rights reserved. No part of the material protected by this copyright may be reproduced or utilized in any form, electronic or mechanical, including photocopying, recording, or by any information storage and retrieval system, without written permission from the copyright owner.

This publication is designed to provide accurate and authoritative information in regard to the subject matter covered. It is sold with the understanding that the publisher is not engaged in rendering legal, accounting, or other professional service. If legal advice or other expert assistance is required, the service of a competent professional person should be sought.

Production Credits
Chief Executive Officer: Ty Field
President: James Homer
SVP, Chief Operating Officer: Don Jones, Jr.
SVP, Chief Technology Officer: Dean Fossella
SVP, Chief Marketing Officer: Alison M. Pendergast
SVP, Chief Financial Officer: Ruth Siporin
Publisher: Michael Brown
Acquisitions Editor: Katey Birtcher
Production Director: Amy Rose
Associate Production Editor: Tina Chen
Marketing Manager: Sophie Fleck
Cover Design: John Garland
Manufacturing and Inventory Control Supervisor: Amy Bacus
Cover Image: © Clockwise, from top: © Julián Rovagnati/ShutterStock, Inc.; © LiquidLibrary;
    © Paul Hill/Fotolia.com; © Dean Mitchell/ShutterStock, Inc. Back cover: © Dean Mitchell/ShutterStock, Inc.

ISBN: 978-1-4496-2923-6

6048
Printed in the United States of America
15 14 13 12 11   10 9 8 7 6 5 4 3 2 1

Contents

Introduction to Health Care Management

Edited by

Sharon B. Buchbinder, RN, PhD
Professor and Chair
Department of Health Science
Towson University
Towson, MD

Nancy H. Shanks, PhD
Chair, Department of Health Professions
Professor and Coordinator, Health Care Management Program
Metropolitan State College of Denver
Denver, CO

JONES AND BARTLETT PUBLISHERS
Sudbury, Massachusetts
BOSTON   TORONTO   LONDON   SINGAPORE

Strategic Planning

Susan Judd Casciani

LEARNING OBJECTIVES

By the end of this chapter, the student will be able to:

- Describe strategic planning and the strategic planning process;
- Identify healthcare market powers, trends, and potential impact on health services;
- Utilize a situational assessment or SWOT analysis;
- Define the links between market volume forecast, core customers, mission, vision, and values;
- Compare data collection methods and strategy tactical plans; and,
- Identify methods to monitor and control strategy execution.

INTRODUCTION

Every organization needs to be successful over the long term in order to survive. A factor critical to that success lies in how well an organization can plan for the future and tap market opportunities. Strategic planning is the process of identifying a desired future state for an organization and a means to achieve it. Through an ongoing analysis of the organization's operating environment, matched against its internal capabilities, an organization's leadership is able to identify strategies that will drive the organization from its present condition to that desired future state.

Strategic planning in health care has had a relatively short history. As recently as the 1970s, strategic planning in the healthcare industry mainly consisted of planning for new buildings and funding expanding services in response to population growth. With the introduction of the federal Prospective Payment System (PPS) in the 1980s, the field of healthcare strategic planning received a transforming jolt as organizations scrambled to compete in an increasingly demanding environment. The turbulent managed care era of the '80s and '90s only served to further fuel the growth of the field, as the cost of healthcare continually rose faster than the Gross Domestic Product (GDP) and competition among providers intensified. Today, hospitals and other healthcare organizations have come to embrace strategic planning as a valuable tool to evaluate alternative paths and help them prepare for the future. Healthcare managers at all levels need to understand the process of strategic planning, its purpose, benefits and challenges, and the key factors for its success.

PURPOSE AND IMPORTANCE OF STRATEGIC PLANNING

In any organization's operating environment there are forces, both controllable and uncontrollable, that will undoubtedly influence the future success of that organization. Only by identifying these forces and planning for ways to adapt to them can an organization achieve the greatest success. At one extreme, completely ignoring these forces can most certainly lead to organizational death. Although no one can predict the future, one can systematically think about it. Accordingly, the purpose of strategic planning is to identify market forces and how they may affect the organization, and determine an appropriate strategic direction to take that will counteract those forces, and/or tap their potential.

Strategic planning serves to focus the organization and also its resource allocation. At any given point in time, there are multiple, and often competing, initiatives and projects to be undertaken in an organization. By understanding the organization's operating environment and identifying a strategy to reach a desired future state, resources can be allocated appropriately and effectively.

THE PLANNING PROCESS

The **strategic planning process** consists mainly of two interrelated activities: the development of the strategic plan, and execution of the organization's strategy. The development of the plan usually spans a multi-year time horizon (3, 5, or 10 years, for example), and is updated annually. **Strategy execution**, on the other hand, is done on a continuous basis and is the critical factor in management of the organization's strategic intentions, optimally providing continual feedback for the development of any future plans.

Although strategic planning is a dynamic and not linear process, Figure 1-1 attempts to depict a logical progression of the steps undertaken to develop a strategic plan. As shown in Figure 1-1, the **Situational Assessment** provides a foundation for strategy development. This Assessment serves two important functions: to provide a snapshot of how the organization is currently interacting with the market in comparison to its internal capabilities and intended strategic direction, and to identify market opportunities and threats that the organization may want to address in future strategic efforts.

Through development of the Situational Assessment, strategy identification can begin. In this stage, the organization's leadership team uses the information and analyses provided in the Situational Assessment to identify specific strategies that may be worthy of pursuit, either to grow the organization or to protect current areas of strength. Once these strategies have been identified, they must be narrowed down to a manageable number through selection and prioritization, and tactical implementation plans must be created. With the strategic plan completed, operating, marketing, and other supporting plans are developed. Control and monitoring of the plan follows, and is most effectively done on an ongoing basis throughout the year. We will look at each of these stages of strategic planning in more detail; however it is important to keep in mind that strategic planning is not a linear process; the feedback loop depicted in Figure 1-1 shows the critical nature of planning being an ongoing, dynamic process.

SITUATIONAL ASSESSMENT

The Situational Assessment is often referred to as a **SWOT (Strengths, Weaknesses, Opportunities, Threats) Analysis,** as it aims to identify the internal strengths and weaknesses of an organization, along with market opportunities and threats. It includes three distinct but intricately related components: the **Market Assessment,** the **Mission, Vision,** and **Values** of the organization, and the **Internal Assessment.** The development of the Market Assessment may be the most complex and time-consuming section

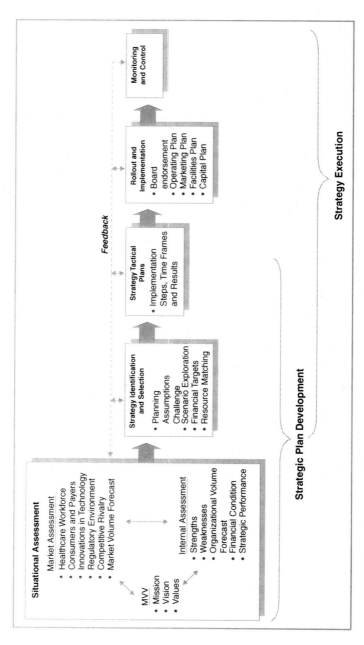

FIGURE 1-1 Strategic Planning Process

of the strategic plan in that, in this section, virtually all aspects of the market must be examined and analyzed to determine their future implications on the organization. Any of a number of market assessment models can be utilized for this analysis, but one of the most common is the **Five Forces Model** developed by Harvard University professor Michael Porter (1998). In this model, Porter identifies five market or industry forces that, when combined, determine the attractiveness of competing in a particular market. For health care, this model can be adapted to analyze the interactions between the **Power of the Healthcare Workforce,** the **Power of Consumers and Payers, Innovations in Technology,** the **Regulatory Environment,** and **Competitive Rivalry.**

The Power of the Healthcare Workforce can have significant strategic implications for any healthcare organization, as its employees act as the frontline caretakers in providing services. In the Market Assessment, an organization should look at the availability of all subsets of healthcare providers that are critical to its success. As an example, if obstetrics is a major clinical program of the organization, the organization should closely consider the future anticipated supply and demand of obstetricians in its market. Currently, with the significant increases in malpractice insurance targeted at obstetricians across the country, many OBs have elected to discontinue delivering babies and focus solely on gynecology, while others have opted to retire early. This has dramatically reduced the supply of obstetricians in many areas of the country, and forced some hospitals to hire their affiliated obstetrical staff in an effort to cover their malpractice insurance premiums and keep them practicing. Other hospitals have developed "laborists"—OBs who are hired solely to work in the hospital and deliver babies. These moves are examples of strategies that could be adopted by organizations to either maintain or grow their obstetrical services in response to market trends.

Another example of the power of the healthcare workforce is the potential ramifications of the current nursing and radiology personnel shortages. With a shortage of personnel, wage and hiring expenses increase, jeopardizing the ability to offer those specific services. A nursing shortage may affect a hospital's ability to add beds to meet growing demand. A shortage of radiology technicians may affect an organization's opportunity to offer new state-of-the-art technologies currently in demand. The influence of these and other healthcare personnel (and the organization's dependency on them) must be considered when developing future strategies.

At the other end of the spectrum are the ultimate purchasers of health care—consumers. The **Power of Consumers** is becoming a more significant market force, and one that has required a dramatic shift in the way the industry offers services. Today's consumers are demanding more and more from their healthcare providers on all levels (e.g. physicians, payers, hospitals, etc.), both in terms of the availability of specific service offerings and in the delivery of those services. For healthcare providers, this has required a shift from the traditional view, where the physician is the primary customer; to today's world, where the patient is the central focus of "customer" service. The potential impact of this shift needs to be considered when developing future strategies.

Consumers can influence the healthcare market in other ways as well. Different communities have different healthcare needs—one community may need increased access to primary care channels, while another may need better health education and screenings. By identifying specific community needs, healthcare organizations can better target their services and potential growth opportunities.

In concert with the Power of Consumers is the **Power of Payers**. Some markets have multiple payers of various sizes and strengths, while others have one or two major payers that dictate market payments. In either case, a healthcare organization that relies on these payers must stay abreast of their needs and demands and how each may affect future operations and strategies. A good example of this is a market with one or two powerful payers where the payers prefer a "late adopter" stance for new medical technologies. In other words, they prefer not to pay for new technologies until the technologies have been proven either medically effective, financially efficient, or both. This would be a significant threat to an organization that strives for a competitive advantage through being first-to-market with the adoption of new medical technologies. The Power of Payers may also create opportunities for an organization. An example would be the general preference of payers for less costly outpatient services. Healthcare organizations that specialize in these types of service offerings (e.g., ambulatory surgery centers, diagnostic/imaging centers) have capitalized on this payer influence in many areas of the country.

The third market power to be considered is **Innovations in Technology**. These innovations may represent the threat of substitute products, as new technologies often replace standard operations and services. A good example of this is the introduction of Picture Archive Communication

Systems (PACs). This filmless imaging system significantly reduces the need for storage space for films and readers and the staff to maintain those areas, as well as allows for remote electronic accessing of files, ultimately requiring a potentially smaller number of physicians necessary to interpret the images. Innovations in technology may also reduce the need for other types of clinical staff, as in the case of some surgical innovations (e.g., minimally invasive surgery, robotic technologies, drug advancements, etc.), and/or they may significantly increase the requirement of financial resources, as in the case of new radiology equipment (e.g., the 64-slice CT scanner, new fluoroscopy equipment, MRI machinery, etc.). As these and other new technologies become available, their potential impact on operations and systems needs to be considered in strategy development.

As the fourth market force, the **Regulatory Environment**—on all levels, federal, state, and local—needs to be monitored for its affects on strategy development as well. Congress continually enacts influential legislation, such as the 1986 Emergency Medical Treatment and Active Labor Act (EMTALA) and the 1996 Health Insurance Portability and Accountability Act (HIPAA), that are indicative of the current focus on mandatory error reporting and physician self-referrals that has significant and rippling effects on all participants in the healthcare industry. Further, the Centers for Medicare and Medicaid Services (CMS) take the lead in changes in healthcare payment formulas that are frequently followed by payers at local levels. Other far-reaching issues, such as liability reform and quality of care measures, may be dealt with on local, state, and federal levels as well. All of these actions can influence a particular healthcare organization's strategy, and need to be monitored and analyzed for their potential impacts.

Competitive Rivalry, the last market force to be considered, is probably given the most significant attention in most organizations' strategy development. Whether an organization operates in a near monopoly or an oligopoly, strategically savvy organizations always track their competitors' moves and suspected intentions. Although it is highly unlikely that you will gain access to the actual strategy of your competitors, much information on their strategic intent can be gleaned from their market activities. Information on their service volumes and market share, as well as news coverage and press releases, should be monitored. Ongoing discussions with the organization's own physicians, staff, and suppliers will likely also yield valuable competitive intelligence. Compiling and synthesizing this information to see a larger picture often leads to an indication of competitors' strategies. Once their strategic intent has been identified, market opportunities for and threats against one's own organization can be further addressed.

Market Volume Forecast

The final component of the Market Assessment is the **Market Volume Forecast**, the purpose of which is to initially develop a quantitative picture of the environment in which the organization will be operating in the future. The forecast is initiated by identifying the organization's service area—usually a zip code-defined area where 70–80% of its patients are drawn from—and determining the population use rates for your applicable service lines (e.g., cardiology, orthopedics, home care visits, CT scans, etc.). These data are usually collected for several historical time periods (e.g. the previous 3 years) and can then be forecasted out several more time periods simply by using a mathematical trend formula, resulting in a base forecast.

For a more realistic forecast, however, assumptions must be overlaid onto this base model. It is critical that the information and data gathered in the market assessment, including the competitor assessment, be incorporated into this forecast in the form of these assumptions. For example, are there new technologies on the horizon that will affect service volumes? Or is there a dearth of providers that may counteract predicted increasing utilization of a particular service for a period of time? Overlaying these assumptions onto the base forecast results in a future scenario for market volume, and any number of future scenarios can be created by adjusting the impacts of the planning assumptions. This is where strategic planning really becomes an art versus a science, and it is often difficult to quantitatively determine the extent to which market forces may affect future market volumes. To this end, there are several companies that provide assistance and/or models for quantifying market forces; a sampling of these companies is provided as additional resources at the end of this chapter.

Mission, Vision, Values

The information gleaned regarding the interaction of these five forces (Healthcare Workforce, Consumers and Payers, Innovations in Technology, Regulatory Environment, and Competitive Rivalry) in the market is matched against the organization's **Mission, Vision,** and **Value (MVV)** statements. As the driving purpose of the organization, the MVVs are reverified as part of the strategic planning process to ensure they continue to be aligned with the organization's future market environment, and to help identify future desired strategic directions. The **Mission** of any organization is its enduring statement of purpose. It aims to identify what the organization does, whom it serves, and how it does it. For example, Radiologix, a radiology services company, "strives to be the premier provider of diagnostic imaging services through high-quality service to patients, referring physicians and mutually beneficial relationships with radiologists who provide expert interpretations of diagnostic images" (http://www .radiologix.com, Retrieved on August 29, 2006). On the other hand, a **Vision statement** strives to identify a specific future state of the organization, usually an inspiring goal for many years down the road. The vision of the American Hospital Association "[is] . . . of a society of healthy communities, where all individuals reach their highest potential for health" (http:// www.aha.org, Retrieved on August 29, 2006). The **Values statement** should help define the organization's culture—what characteristics it wants employees to convey to customers. An example of one such value from Duke University Health System in North Carolina is: "We earn the trust our patients place in us by involving them in their healthcare planning and treatment and by exceeding their service expectations" (http://www.duke health.org/AboutDuke/Mission/mission_statement, Retrieved on August 29, 2006).

Although the mission statement is generally the most enduring of the three, each of these statements may be altered over time to adapt to the environment. As an example, the increasing influence of consumerism in healthcare drove many an organization to revise its vision and value statements to become more customer-service focused, which in turn (hopefully) helped to change the organization's culture. Reaffirming and/or adjusting these three statements in relation to market activity is a critical step in determining the desired future state of the organization.

Internal Assessment

The third component of the Situational Assessment, the **Internal Assessment**, is matched against both the Mission, Vision, and Values Statements and the Market Assessment to complete the situational snapshot. In conducting an internal assessment, an organization turns the analytical lens inward to examine areas of strength and weakness, as well as how it may build or sustain a competitive advantage in the market. Like the Market

Assessment, the Internal Assessment has both quantitative as well as qualitative components. The quantitative section of the internal assessment consists mainly of the organizational volume forecast and an assessment of the financial condition. The qualitative section focuses on past strategic performance, and leadership's interpretation of the organization's core capabilities (or lack thereof).

Organizational Volume Forecast

The **Organizational Volume Forecast** takes the base model forecast developed in the market assessment and applies historical market share information, therein highlighting some of an organization's strengths and weaknesses. By holding its market share growth trends constant in the future scenarios, an organization can formulate a preliminary idea of how well it would fare if it (and its competitors) were to stay its current course. Examining the forecast from the perspective of market share, contribution margin, and/or medical staff depth will also yield service lines of strength that may need to be protected, as well as service lines that could be developed further.

As with the development of the previous future scenarios however, it is important to apply assumptions to the forecasts. For example, will the organization plan to hold market share constant for a particular service, or will the organization hope to grow that market? Alternately, the organization may decide to discontinue a specific service, perhaps due to predicted declining reimbursements or lack of physicians. It is important to keep in mind that any alternative scenarios that are created will be used as input for the development of specific strategies in the next phase of the planning process, at which time their underlying planning assumptions should be debated extensively.

Financial Condition

As with the volume forecast, several years' worth of **key financial indicators** should be analyzed to highlight additional strengths and weaknesses of the organization. These may include indicators such as operating margin, net income, gross and net revenues, bond ratings, fund raising, key financial ratios, payer mix, pricing and/or rate setting arrangements. The organization's historical performance against budget is also helpful to analyze, and should yield further insight into strengths and weaknesses. Any financial forecasts that are available should also be included, as well as any routine or planned capital spending and/or facility improvement plans. It is critical to tie the financial reserves and needs of the organization to the strategic planning process to ensure the resulting strategies can and will be funded appropriately. Tying the financial information to the volume forecast also serves to provide budget targets for the upcoming year(s).

Strategic Performance

It is important to remember that, as mentioned earlier, strategic planning is a dynamic rather than a linear process and as such there should optimally be no distinct beginning or end. Thus, a review of the organization's past strategic performance should be included as part of future strategy development. This review can be as simple as an assessment of whether past strategies accomplished intended goals, or as multifaceted as an ad hoc leadership meeting to discuss roadblocks that led to failure or factors that drove success. Either way, this review can and should provide valuable information for future strategy development and implementation.

Leadership Input

In addition to the more quantitative strengths and weaknesses outlined through the volume forecast and financial condition review, there are subjective strengths and weaknesses that need to be identified for strategy development as well. Identifying these capabilities can be quite challenging, as planners usually have to rely on surveys of and/or interviews with the leadership of the organization to gather this information. This can be both time consuming and value laden, but this information will be critical input for the plan's overall success. With that said, Table 1-1 highlights some common methods of collecting this information, and the benefits and limitations of each.

The key to gathering the most value from the leadership input is to challenge leaders (e.g., executives, physicians, managers, etc.) to think within a strategic context, as opposed to the operational mode they are involved in on a day-to-day basis. Merely asking leaders to identify an organization's weaknesses, for example, can result in responses such as parking or a lack of marketing, whereas framing the question to identify challenges to the organization in growing service volumes may better yield answers such as an aging medical staff, lack of capacity, etc. It is important to incorporate these identified strengths and weaknesses into the Internal Assessment for further discussion.

TABLE 1-1 Data Collection Methods

	Pros	Cons
Interviews	■ Opportunity to clarify responses ■ Encourages free thinking ■ Can ensure representative sample	■ Time consuming ■ Potential for interviewer bias ■ Open answers difficult to analyze
Focus Groups	■ Opportunity to clarify responses ■ Allows for relatively large sample ■ Can be economically efficient	■ Potential for groupthink ■ Open answers difficult to analyze
Surveys	■ Effective way to obtain large sample ■ Standardized answers allow for easier analysis ■ No interviewer bias	■ Can be expensive ■ Lag time for responses ■ Potential for low response rate

Strategy Identification and Selection

Throughout the development and analyses of the overall Situational Assessment, the building blocks for strategy identification begin to emerge. If the organization is at the start of the development of a multi-year plan, it will usually conduct a rather thorough Situational Assessment. However, if the organization has an identified long-term strategic direction, the Situational Assessment may selectively analyze only those areas that are relevant to the identified strategic direction. For example, if the organization has resolved to grow defined service lines, the assessment may focus more specifically on those areas of the market. Alternately, if the direction is diversification, the assessment may focus more on areas related to the organization's current strengths, whether they are service line or internal capability related. Regardless of the depth of the Situational Assessment, it serves as input for the next step in the process, **Strategy Identification** and **Selection.**

With the backdrop of the Situational Assessment, strategy identification begins by analyzing and challenging the planning assumptions, further exploring any future scenarios developed earlier, and incorporating any desired financial targets as determined by leadership. From this analysis, several potential strategic directions for the organization may emerge. The strategic direction is the goal that the organization desires to accomplish within the planning timeframe. Generally, as each direction may have different probabilities for success and require different levels of resource investment, the specific direction that will ultimately be chosen will often depend on an organization's tolerance for risk.

Once a strategic direction is chosen, specific desired outcomes should be targeted and strategies identified to accomplish it. As an example, if an organization concludes it will differentiate itself through its orthopedic services (strategic direction), the desired outcome may be to lead the market in orthopedic service volumes within two years. To accomplish this, the organization may identify strategies to increase its surgeon base, add rehabilitation services, or develop a center of excellence program. A strategy is a carefully designed plan to accomplish the desired outcomes.

Even the largest and most fiscally sound organization cannot successfully implement all the strategies it can conceive of, nor should it try to. A successful strategic plan is focused and, just as importantly, executable; too many strategies may render the plan ineffective simply because there is too much to do. Strategy is all about making choices. A clear and focused strategy will guide decision making, prioritize resource allocation and keep the organization on its desired course; in choosing which strategies to pursue, an organization is also choosing which strategies not to pursue. At this stage in the planning process, the organization's leadership must determine its ability to successfully execute the strategies it has identified.

Factors to consider in making this determination include the degree to which the strategy has the ability to help the organization meet its financial targets. Alternately, does the organization have the financial resources to fund the strategy appropriately in terms of operating and capital expense? Additionally, does the organization have the internal capabilities to successfully execute the strategy—does it have, or can it acquire, the necessary human resources? Is the strategy transformational enough to bring about the desired change? Equally important, is there a champion to take ownership of the strategy's success? By going through the exercise of matching potential strategies to financial and other targets, and matching implementation requirements to resource availability, strategy selection is accomplished (see Table 1-2).

STRATEGY TACTICAL PLANS

The final step in the actual development of the strategic plan is the creation of specific tactical plans for each strategy, which are necessary for translating the plan into action.

TABLE 1-2 **Successful Strategies**

Successful strategies:

- Are focused on the desired future state
- Align internal capabilities with market opportunities and threats
- Provide or sustain a competitive advantage for the organization
- Are funded and resourced long term

Tactical plans answer the who, what, when, where, and how questions of strategy implementation. Table 1-3 shows an example of a basic template for a tactical plan that, when completed, will help drive implementation of the strategy.

ROLLOUT AND IMPLEMENTATION

With the development of the tactical plans, the strategic plan is complete. The plan is then presented to the Board of Directors for approval and endorsement, and is then rolled out across the organization. **Rollout** of the plan has two main steps: first, the plan is communicated at all levels of the organization; only by communicating the strategy to all necessary stakeholders can an organization gain the support necessary for successful execution of the strategy.

Second, supporting plans such as the financial and budgeting plans, operating plan, marketing plan, capital plan, and master facilities plan are developed or updated with the intent and strategies developed in the strategic plan. Having all of the organization's supporting plans tied to the

TABLE 1-3 **Tactical Plan Template**

Goal	Key Actions	Target Completion Date	Resources Required	Dependencies	Revenue Projection	Success Metric

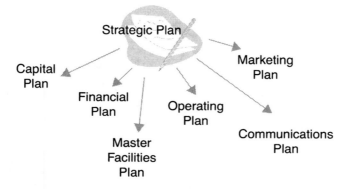

FIGURE 1-2 Supporting Plans

strategic plan is a critical factor in reinforcing its strategic direction. Figure 1-2 depicts some of the supporting plans that may be drawn from the strategic plan.

MONITORING AND CONTROL

Monitoring and control of the strategic plan is most often accomplished through the use of an **organizational dashboard,** or **scorecard.** A dashboard is a visual reference used to monitor an organization's performance against targets over time. Its simplistic design should allow for quick assessment of areas that may need adjustment, similar to an automobile dashboard. Dashboards can depict strategic, operational and/or financial indicators, depending on the organization's needs, but care must be taken to highlight a manageable number of indicators or the dashboard will lose its functionality. Figure 1-3 depicts an example of a dashboard, although many other templates abound in the industry.

Depending on the organization's needs, and depending on the types of indicators management identifies, the dashboard should be monitored regularly (e.g. monthly or quarterly). At a minimum, as soon as an indicator highlights a variance from the desired target, managers must address the variance with tactics that correct or alter the results, but optimally, the dashboard should serve to facilitate management discussion regarding execution of the strategy. To best ensure success of the strategic plan, dashboard indicators are aligned with operational plans and their associated identified goals.

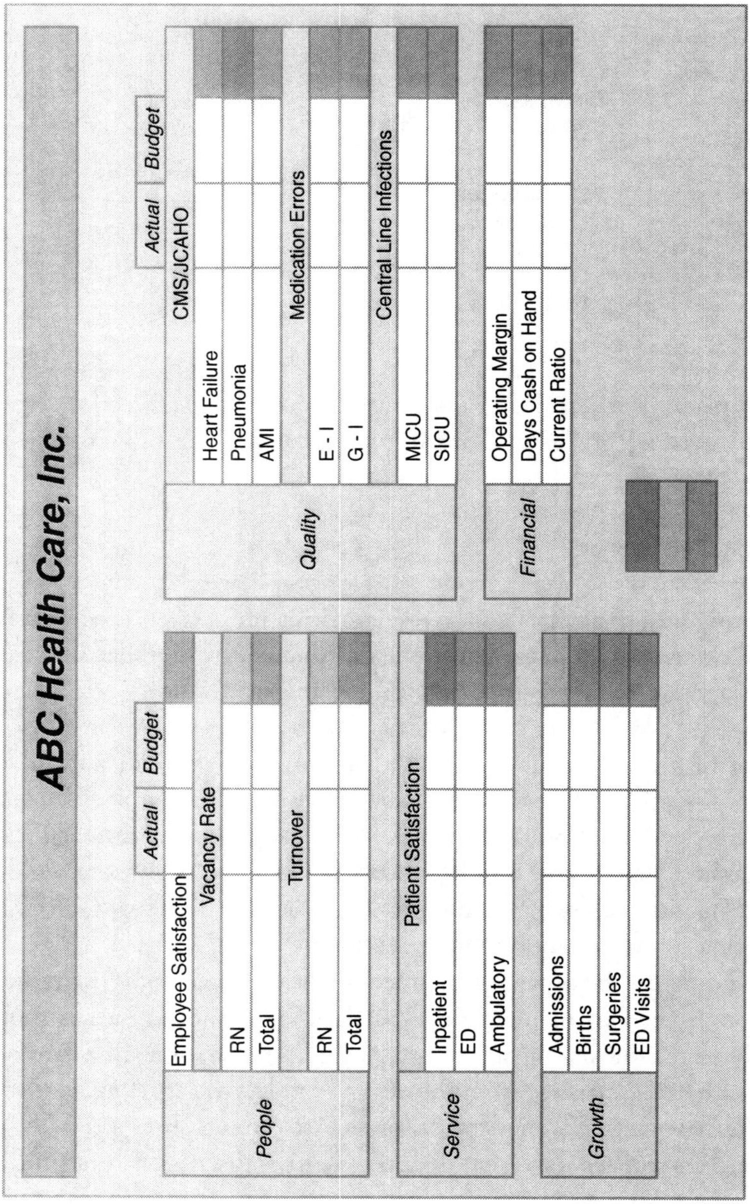

FIGURE 1-3 Dashboard

STRATEGY EXECUTION

Although the development of the actual strategic plan occurs in a logical progression, other than perhaps the creation of the Situational Assessment, every stage of the plan's development should be viewed as part of its execution. **Strategy execution** is crucial for organizational success and cannot be overstated in terms of importance. Unfortunately, this is often an element of strategic planning that many organizations overlook. With the flurry of activity and intensity that usually surrounds the development of the strategic plan itself, there can be a collective sigh of relief following board approval of the plan, and leadership may be relieved to be able to return to their "real work" and the day-to-day operations. Yet successful organizations know that execution is much more important than the plan.

Execution, however, isn't easy and there are many roadblocks on the path to success. For example, it has been said that "culture eats strategy for lunch," and even that may be an understatement. If an organization's stakeholders are not ready for the strategy, it will not be executed by even the most tenacious of leaders. With the heightened influence of consumerism, many healthcare organizations attempted strategies early on to shift the organization from a more physician-centric to a patient-centric focus, aiming to gain a competitive advantage on this emerging market trend. However, many of these same organizations were faced with a strong undercurrent of resistance from an internal culture that was not prepared for this new paradigm, and the strategy failed. This example demonstrates the need for strategy execution to start early in the planning process, enabling the organization to either better prepare itself for implementation of the strategy or to table the strategy until the organization is ready to implement it successfully.

Other barriers to successful strategy execution include a lack of strategic focus. Often during the plan development phase, leadership will inevitably develop more strategies than it can successfully execute. If this list is not pared down to a reasonable number, or if the few strategies that are planned do not align appropriately, execution attempts will be futile. Additionally, as mentioned earlier, if the strategies are not appropriately funded and resourced they cannot be executed, or if they result in competing priorities, the organization will likely be unsuccessful. All of these barriers can be overcome, however, in part by focusing on execution at the earliest stages of strategy development.

Strategy execution is also most successful with a combination of strong leadership and organizational buy-in. Although leadership will need to have flexibility to adjust strategies as market conditions warrant, they must also have the consistency over time to stay the course. Too often, strategies have failed because an organization has fallen to the temptation of new priorities, or has simply neglected to resource the strategy over multiple years or time periods. Strategy is not a quick fix nor does it promise immediate turnaround; strong leadership is needed to maintain a long-term focus. In addition, organizational buy-in at all levels is critical. As demonstrated earlier in the example regarding culture, strategy cannot be implemented solely in the top layers of an organization. All stakeholders must be aware of and buy into the desired future state and the path that leads them there in order to ensure the momentum necessary to achieve results. Optimally, a successfully conducted strategic planning process will generate strategy champions at all levels of the organization.

Participants

All organizations generally involve key leadership in the strategic planning process, but the extent to which other stakeholders are involved varies considerably. There is no one best answer as to who should be involved in the planning process and how as each organization and culture is different, but one caveat generally always holds true: the more stakeholders that are aware of and own the strategy, the greater the chance of success. That said, the strategic planning process should involve representatives from the Board of Trustees, upper and middle management, the medical staff, general staff, and community leaders throughout the process, as much as is feasible. When the plan is completed, it should be communicated to all stakeholders as discussed earlier.

STRATEGIC PLANNING AND EXECUTION— THE ROLE OF THE HEALTHCARE MANAGER

A good portion of this chapter has been dedicated to discussion of the content of the strategic plan, and with good reason—healthcare managers need to understand the types of information and intelligence gathered and analyzed for plan development, and how that information is interpreted and acted upon. However, it has often been said that the plan is worthless, but planning is priceless; the value of strategic planning lies not in the plan itself, but in the planning process. Properly conducted, the strategic planning process will challenge management to robustly confront the brutal facts of its market and the organization, to persistently test planning assumptions, and to continually refine the organization's execution skills.

Healthcare managers at all levels have the responsibility to continually monitor their environment—both internal and external—and assess and act upon the possible implications of any trends or events that are of note. They have the responsibility to understand their local market on an ongoing basis and to know their organization's strategic direction and intent. They are responsible for identifying ways to support the organization's strategy, and for ensuring that their subordinates have the knowledge and understanding of the strategy in order to do the same. Strategic planning may be driven by the planning or business development function of an organization, but it is the responsibility of leadership at all levels to help execute and manage the organization's strategy.

CONCLUSION

Effective strategic planning is a critical element in the success of today's healthcare organizations. Through understanding its competitive and other market environments, an organization can best identify a desired future state and a means to achieve it, but as discussed, the true value of strategic planning lies in the process, and less in the resulting plan. In a recent study, Begun and Kaissi (2005) investigated the perceived value of strategic planning to leaders in 20 healthcare organizations. Consistent with the information presented in this chapter, the authors found that leadership stressed the dynamic versus static nature of planning, and the importance of execution of the strategic plan. Strategic planning will likely continue to be a valued function in healthcare organizations in the future, and management at all levels needs to understand the process and its purpose, and its role in development and execution of the successful strategy.

DISCUSSION QUESTIONS

1. What are some of the healthcare market trends you can identify in your market? How might they affect your job as a manager, and how would you react to/prepare for them?

2. In what ways can you, as a manager, contribute to the management and execution of your organization's strategy?

3. Discuss how strategic planning is a dynamic, versus linear, process. Why is this important?

4. What is the purpose of the Situational Assessment, and how is it best used in the planning process?

REFERENCES

Begun, J. & Kaissi, A. (2005). An exploratory study of healthcare strategic planning in two metropolitan areas. *Journal of Healthcare Management, 50*(4), 264–274.

Porter, M. (1998). *On competition.* Cambridge, MA: Harvard Business School Publishing.

Additional Readings

Bossidy, L., & Charan, R. (2004). Execution: the discipline of getting things done. *AFP Exchange, 24*(1), 26–30.

Brandenburger, A., & Nalebuff, B. (1995). The right game: use game theory to shape strategy. *Harvard Business Review, 73*(4), 57–71.

Collins, J. (2001). *Good to great: why some companies make the leap . . . and others don't.* New York: Harper Business.

Collis, D., & Montgomery, C. (1995). Competing on resources: strategy in the 1990's. *Harvard Business Review, 73*(4), 118–129.

Ginter, P., Swayne, L., & Duncan, W. J. (2002). *Strategic management of healthcare organizations (4th ed.).* Malden, MA: Blackwell Publishers, Inc.

Jennings, M. (Ed.). (2000). *Health care strategy for uncertain times.* San Francisco, CA: Jossey-Bass.

Kaplan, R., & Norton, D. (1996). *The balanced scorecard: translating strategy into action.* Cambridge, MA: Harvard Business School Publishing.

Kaplan, R., & Norton, D. (2005). The balanced scorecard: measures that drive performance. *Harvard Business Review, 83*(7), 172.

Prahalad, C. K., & Ramaswamy, V. (2004). *The future of competition: co-creating unique value with customers.* Cambridge, MA: Harvard Business School Publishing.

Senge, P., Kleiner, A., Roberts, C., Ross, R. B., Roth, G., & Smith, B. J. (1994). *The fifth discipline fieldbook: strategies and tools for building a learning organization.* New York: Doubleday.

Zuckerman, A. (2005). Creating competitive advantage: product development. *Healthcare Financial Management, 59*(6), 110–113.

Additional Websites to Explore

Sg2	www.sg2.com
Solucient	www.solucient.com
Data Bay Resources	www.databayresources.com
The Advisory Board Company	www.advisoryboardcompany.com

CHAPTER 2

Performance Improvement in Health Care: The Quest to Achieve Quality

Grant T. Savage
Eric S. Williams

LEARNING OBJECTIVES

By the end of this chapter the student will be able to:

- Define healthcare quality from a variety of stakeholder perspectives;
- Discuss the importance of quality to a healthcare system;
- Trace the evolution of quality thinking, from quality assurance to continuous quality improvement to systems improvement;
- Describe the leading models of quality improvement;
- Define and apply key quality concepts; and,
- Describe and discuss four future challenges.

INTRODUCTION

Cost, access, and quality form the health policy triumvirate. Quality, as a key policy consideration, gained significant public focus in the United States with two recent publications by the Institute of Medicine (IOM): *To*

Err is Human (Kohn, Corrigan, & Donaldson, 2000) and *Crossing the Quality Chasm* (Institute of Medicine, 2001). *Too Err is Human* is the IOM report that first brought public attention to the issue of medical errors, concluding that between 44,000 and 98,000 people die every year from these errors. It also diagnosed the quality problem as not one of poorly performing people, but of people struggling to perform within a system riddled with opportunities for mistakes—known as latent errors— waiting to happen. The second IOM report, *Crossing the Quality Chasm*, outlines a number of goals for improving the quality and performance of the United States healthcare system, as well as some of the methods for achieving those goals.

This chapter builds on these two significant reports. The first two sections describe several of the more common definitions of quality and present the case for the importance of quality as the ultimate measure of performance for healthcare organizations. The third section examines the historical evolution of quality thinking in health care, from initial conceptions of quality assurance in the 19th century to the adoption of continuous quality improvement in the 1980s and 1990s. The fourth section presents the leading models of quality currently used in health care, while the fifth section expands on some of the key quality concepts that underlie many of the quality models discussed in the text. The sixth section traces the emergence of system improvement and system thinking during the turn of the 21st century, while the final section presents a number of quality and performance challenges that appear on the horizon for patients, policy makers, and providers.

DEFINING QUALITY IN HEALTH CARE

Healthcare quality may be defined in various ways, with differing implications for healthcare providers, patients, third-party payers, policy makers, and other stakeholders. In what follows, we examine the leading definitions and some of their implications for stakeholders. The National Academies' Institute of Medicine (IOM) provides the most widely accepted definition of healthcare quality as the "degree to which health services for individuals or populations increase the likelihood of desired health outcomes and are consistent with the current professional knowledge" (Institute of Medicine, 1990). This definition highlights several aspects of quality. First, high quality health services should achieve desired health outcomes for individuals, matching their preferences for variety. Second, they should achieve desired health outcomes for populations, matching the societal preferences of policy makers and third-party payers for efficiency. And, third, they should adhere to professional standards and scientific evidence, consistent with the clinical focus and preferences of healthcare providers for effectiveness.

Another way to view quality is as the result of a system with interdependent parts that must work together to achieve outcomes such as those noted above. Avedis Donabedian, a physician who was a leading advocate for improving healthcare quality during the last half of the 20th century, introduced the idea that quality could be viewed from a system perspective as structure, processes, and outcomes (Donabedian, 1966). The structural elements of quality involve the material and human resources of an organization and the facility itself. Simply put, this is the quality of the setting and the people, whether in a hospital, physician's office, nursing home, or hospice. Processes are the actual activities of patient care and all the ancillary activities attending the interaction between patients and providers. Outcomes are the resulting health status of the patients. As a physician, Donabedian championed the development of "best practices" to achieve better care (Cooper, 1999), linking structures, processes, and outcomes with a feedback loop. Moreover, he defined quality as having at least four components (Donabedian, 1986):

1. The technical management of health and illness
2. The management of the interpersonal relationship between the providers of care and their clients
3. The amenities of care
4. The ethical principles that govern the conduct of affairs in general and the healthcare enterprise in particular.

The four parts of this definition highlight the need to incorporate multiple stakeholder perspectives to understand healthcare quality. On one hand, the technical management of health focuses on the clinical performance of healthcare providers; on the other hand, the management of interpersonal relationships underscores the co-production of care by both providers and patients. In other words, at the patient-provider encounter level, health service quality is driven both by clinical and non-clinical processes (Marley, Collier, & Goldstein, 2004). The "amenities of care" speak to patients' interest in pursuing individual well-being (or variety);

the "ethical principles" speak to providers' interests in furthering societal and organizational well-being (or effectiveness).

A related and more focused view of quality represents two fundamental questions about any clinical service, procedure, or activity occurring in a healthcare setting: 1) "Are the right things done?" and 2) "Are things done right?" The first question assesses the effectiveness of clinical care; the second considers the efficiency of care services. Importantly, the performance of healthcare organizations depends on their effectiveness and their efficiency. Moreover, both effectiveness and efficiency are discussed in the IOM's *Crossing the Quality Chasm* as two of six specific aims for quality improvement. Effectiveness is defined as "providing services based on scientific knowledge to all who could benefit and refraining from providing services to those not likely to benefit (avoiding underuse and overuse)"; efficiency is defined as "avoiding waste, in particular waste of equipment, supplies, ideas, and energy" (Institute of Medicine, 2001).

WHY IS QUALITY IMPORTANT?

One of the key issues in healthcare quality and performance is the appropriate use of scarce resources to improve the health of both individuals and the entire population. Problems in this domain can take three forms: underuse, overuse, and misuse. Chassin (1997) defines these terms as follows:

> [**Underuse** is] the failure to provide a service whose benefit is greater than its risk. **Overuse** occurs when a health service is provided when its risks outweigh its benefits. **Misuse** occurs when the right service is provided badly and an avoidable complication reduces the benefit the patient receives.

Underuse is a problem since clinical research has produced a large number of proven, effective treatments that are not widely used. For example, beta blockers are effective in preventing heart attacks among patients who previously have had a heart attack. A study in the late 1990s found that only 21% of eligible elderly patients were prescribed beta blockers upon release after their first heart attack (Soumerai, McLaughlin, Spiegelman, Hertzmark, Thibault, & Goldman, 1997). More recent studies suggest that the underuse of beta blockers, not only in the United States but also in other parts of the world, may occur because of hospital- and clinician-based prescribing patterns (Fonarow, 2005; Nicholls, McElduff, Dobson, Jamrozik, Hobbs, & Leitch, 2001).

Overuse is also a quality problem, as certain treatments are provided despite evidence that the treatment is ineffective or, even, dangerous. Gonzales, Steiner, and Sande (1997) document the overuse of antibiotics among their sample of adults. They found that antibiotics were prescribed 51% of the time for common colds, 52% for upper respiratory infections, and 75% for bronchitis. Such prescriptions are written even though these maladies are caused by viruses, not bacteria. Further, the indiscriminant use of antibiotics has fed the rise of multi-drug resistant strains of bacteria (Steinberg, 2000).

Misuse caught the public's attention with the publication of the first IOM report on patient safety, *To Err is Human* (Kohn, Corrigan, & Donaldson, 2000), which examined the high rate of medical errors in hospitals, noting that between 44,000 and 98,000 hospitalized patients die each year from preventable adverse events and a further 1,000,000 are injured. Moreover, the IOM estimated that the costs to the U.S. economy totaled between $37.6 to $50 billion dollars each year in 1999. Importantly, these figures only represent inpatient, hospital-based services. Recent studies estimate that 3.5% to 6% of outpatients will experience moderate to serious adverse drug events. Solberg and his colleagues used four years of claims data to identify potential drug-drug interactions that alter the effectiveness or toxicity of one or more drugs (Solberg, Hurley, Roberts, Nelson, Frost, Crain, Gunter, & Young, 2004). They found that about 3.5% of those prescribed drugs are at risk in any given year for moderate to severe drug-drug interactions. Using a different methodology of chart auditing and patient surveys, Gandhi and his colleagues reported that 6% of outpatients experienced adverse drug events that were either serious and preventable or ameliorable (Gandhi, Weingart, Borus, Seger, Peterson, Burdick, Seger, Shu, Federico, Leape, & Bates, 2003).

The *Dartmouth Atlas of Health Care* (see http://www.dartmouthatlas.org/) illustrates the prevalence of healthcare service underuse, overuse, and misuse in the United States. The atlas, created by John Wennberg and his associates, captures and displays wide variations in medical practice that cannot be explained by illness severity or patient preference. The pattern of these variations is "often idiosyncratic and unscientific, and local medical opinion and local supply of resources are more important than science in determining how medical care is delivered" (Wennberg, 2002). For example, Boston and New Haven are demographically similar, geographically close, and might be expected to be fairly similar in their utilization of surgical services. However, residents of New Haven were "more than twice as likely to receive coronary bypass surgery and 50% more likely to undergo hysterectomy" than Bostonians. In addition, Bostonians "were two times more likely to undergo carotid artery surgery and 50% more likely to have their hip joints replaced than the residents of New Haven" (Wennberg, 2002).

A BRIEF HISTORY OF QUALITY AND PERFORMANCE IMPROVEMENT

While healthcare policy makers in the United States and other industrialized countries have recently focused their attention on quality, both patients and the providers of health services have valued it for countless millennia. For example, the Codex Hammurabi (circa 1700 BC) imposes several forms of punishment—including death—to physicians and nurses providing poor quality care (Spiegel & Springer, 1997). Similarly, the Hippocratic Oath (circa 400 BC) admonishes physicians to keep patients from "harm or injustice" (von Staden, 1996). Modern versions of the oath continue to be adhered to by physicians and to be incorporated into medical training (Smith, 1996), evolving during the past century into a professional code of ethics (Davis, 2003). Even though the concern about healthcare quality has a long history, its connection to performance improvement is much more recent, arising during the second half of the 19th century and continuing today. The modern history of quality and performance improvement in healthcare services can be divided into three relatively distinct eras: Quality Assurance (QA), Continuous Quality Improvement (CQI), and Systems Improvement (SI). We are now immersed in this latter era, but the techniques and practices of QA and CQI remain and are the basis for improving the system of health care in the United States and around the world.

QUALITY ASSURANCE

The beginnings of the quality assurance era can be traced to the mid-19th century, about the same time as the scientific understanding of germ-induced illness was gaining support in Europe. For most healthcare practitioners, quality assurance is associated with the observations and reforms made by Florence Nightingale during the Crimean War of 1854. During her service as a nurse, she noted a correlation between poor hospital sanitation and an alarming rate of fatalities among wounded soldiers. Acting on this observation, she developed hospital sanitation and hygiene standards during the war that sharply decreased mortality and morbidity rates. Nightingale promoted such basic precautions as washing hands, cleaning surgical tools, providing fresh bed linens, and ensuring hospital wards were clean. During the remainder of the 19th century, she devoted her life to a reform movement that significantly upgraded the practices of sanitation and hygiene in hospitals, while also significantly improving the training of nurses and expanding their role in health care (Henry, Woods, & Nagelkerk, 1990).

THE END RESULT SYSTEM AND THE FLEXNER REPORT

Building upon Nightingale's precepts, Ernest Codman, a Harvard Medical School surgeon, advocated that hospitals should examine whether the services provided to patients were beneficial and address the reasons for failure. His "End Result System" was introduced in 1910, and articulated three core principles of quality assurance: 1) examining quality measures to determine if problems are patient-, system-, or clinician-related; 2) assessing the frequency and prevalence of quality deficiencies; and 3) evaluating and correcting deficiencies so that they do not reoccur (Cooper, 1999). By 1917, the End Result System was acknowledged as critical to ensuring quality health care, and it became the basis for the Hospitalization Standardization Program of the American College of Surgeons. This program established "minimum standards" that focused on the quality of care within hospitals, including the 1) organizing of hospital medical staffs; 2) restricting of medical staff membership to well-trained, competent, and licensed physicians; 3) framing of policies and procedures to ensure regular staff meetings and clinical reviews; 4) recording of medical histories, physical exams, and laboratory tests; and 5) developing diagnostic and treatment facilities under physician oversight (Luce, Bindman, & Lee, 1994). When the American College of Surgeons began on-site inspections of hospitals in 1918, only 89 of 692 hospitals surveyed met minimum standards; by 1950, more than 3,200 hospitals were approved under the Hospitalization Standardization Program (JCAHO, 2006).

About the same time as Codman set forth his ideas, a committee headed by Abraham Flexner was investigating the quality of medical education in

North America for the Carnegie Foundation. His committee's report, *Medical Education in the United States and Canada*, was published in 1910 (Flexner, 1972, c1910). The report strongly criticized proprietary medical schools, including homeopathic and osteopathic approaches, and faulted their poor apprenticeship system. To improve medical education, the committee endorsed biomedical studies in biology, chemistry, and physics that were integrated with rigorous clinical training. The Flexner report revolutionized medical education, supplanting many other forms of physician education with the biomedical model, and integrating it with supervised clinical training. Both Codman and Flexner advanced the science of medical practice, laying the groundwork for future health professionals' acceptance and participation in quality assurance activities.

THE JOINT COMMISSION

In 1951, the American College of Physicians, the American Hospital Association, the American Medical Association, the Canadian Medical Association, and the American College of Surgeons created the Joint Commission on the Accreditation of Hospitals (JCAH). The Joint Commission was formed as a not-for-profit organization to provide voluntary accreditation to hospitals. The American College of Surgeons' Hospital Standardization Program—inspired by Codman's End Result System—was adopted as JCAH's accreditation tool, and the ACS officially transferred this program to the Joint Commission in 1952, and began surveying hospitals in 1953 (JCAHO, 2006). Although the Canadian Medical Association withdrew from the Joint Commission in 1959 in order to establish a Canadian accrediting body, the American Dental Association became a corporate member in 1979 (Viswanathan & Salmon, 2000).

With the passage of legislation authorizing Medicare and Medicaid in 1965, the Joint Commission grew in importance. The legislation contained a provision that JCAH accredited hospitals were deemed to be in compliance with most of the Medicare Conditions of Participation for Hospitals and, thus, could participate in the Medicare and Medicaid programs (JCAHO, 2006; Sprague, 2005). On one hand, this provision made the accreditation process much more compelling to hospital administrators. On the other hand, it meant a change in focus for the Joint Commission's quality assurance approach, from ensuring that minimum standards were followed by hospitals to one based on optimal achievable standards (Luce, Bindman, & Lee 1994). It also marked the beginning of the expansion of the Joint Commission's scope of accreditation. In 1966 it began accrediting long-term facilities; psychiatric facilities, substance abuse programs, and community mental health programs in 1970; ambulatory healthcare facilities in 1975; and hospice organizations in 1983. Thus, it was not surprising that in 1987, the Joint Commission changed its formal name to the Joint Commission on Accreditation of Healthcare Organizations (JCAHO) to reflect its expanded scope of activities beyond hospital accreditation (JCAHO, 2002).

QA ESSENTIALS

As the Joint Commission expanded its scope and activities from the 1950s to the 1980s, the End Result System evolved into Quality Assurance (QA). Essentially, QA involves the development of standards, and the measurement of individual, group, or organizational performance against such standards. In terms of Donabedian's structure-process-outcome framework (Donabedian, 1966), most QA standards focus on structural variables, with some recognition of process and outcome variables. Indeed, until the 1990s, the Joint Commission tended to focus on structural standards, such as assuring that a hospital's physicians were board certified, its nurses licensed, and other key employees had appropriate certifications (Gilpatrick, 1999). It also assured that a hospital had the appropriate numbers and quality of items (e.g., beds, surgical equipment) and appropriate policies and procedures.

Critical to the operation of these standards is the function of tracking and trending. Tracking begins with the identification and monitoring of indicators that reflect standards of care. Benchmarking is often used to identify clinical indicators and "best practices" associated with each. For instance, beginning in 2002, the JCAHO has required hospitals to measure quality of care indicators for the following illnesses: acute myocardial infarction, heart failure, pneumonia, and pregnancy. Care indicators associated with each of these illnesses were identified through an intensive process of reviewing clinical studies and conferring with expert panels of physicians. Field tests of the indicators resulted in four sets of validated measures (Williams, Schmaltz, Morton, Koss, & Loeb, 2005). A few examples of quality of care measures for acute myocardial infarction (heart attack) include aspirin and beta-blocker within 24 hours of admission and smoking-cessation counseling. Indicators such as these are then monitored at repeated intervals, requiring extensive data collection by trained individuals familiar with the measurement process. Gathering data for many clinical process indicators now requires that hospital or medical group personnel abstract data from patient charts. However, the increased use of electronic medical records should eventually automate this process, while prompting physicians to employ best practices (Delpierre, Cuzin, Fillaux, Alvarez, Massip, & Lang, 2004; Rubenfeld, 2004).

QA ASSUMPTIONS AND ACTIONS

From a QA perspective, once sufficient data is gathered, there are two possible outcomes. The first is that the healthcare provider meets or exceeds the standard. When this outcome occurs, no action needs to take place. However, if a provider does not meet the standard for a measure, then the responsible party for QA—a medical director, quality assurance department, or regulatory agency—must take action. The book, *Forgive and Remember: Managing Medical Failure* (Bosk, 1979), portrays the surgical culture of personal accountability upon which QA is grounded, and underscores QA's core assumption that people are responsible for most medical errors. Hence, the responsible party will identify those individuals, groups, or organizations causing the poor performance. Those associated with the quality deficiency will then face one of several responses, depending on the severity of the deficiency. They may be required to attend educational or retraining sessions, provided with technical assistance, and/or be disciplined. For individual providers, disciplinary actions may lead to the revocation of their licenses to practice; for organizations, certification or operating licenses may be rescinded.

At the same time that the Joint Commission was refining the practices associated with QA, the federal government was committed to assuring the quality of services provided to Medicare and Medicaid recipients. Moreover, both the Joint Commission and the Health Care Financing Administration (HCFA)—now known as the Centers for Medicare and Medicaid Services (CMS)—gradually moved away from QA to CQI approaches for improving healthcare quality. How and why these changes took place is discussed next.

FROM PEER REVIEW TO QUALITY IMPROVEMENT ORGANIZATIONS

The introduction of Medicare and Medicaid in 1965 dramatically changed the role and responsibilities of the federal government in the United States. Because Medicare and Medicaid were providing health insurance to a substantial portion of the population, Congress demanded assurance that public funds were being spent for both medically necessary and quality services and items. Initially, Congress authorized the Experimental Medical Care Review Organizations (EMCRO) in 1971. The EMCRO reviewed inpatient and ambulatory services for appropriateness and quality of care, establishing the model for the Professional Standards Review Organizations (PSRO) that would soon follow (Bhatia, Blackstock, Nelson, & Ng, 2000).

PROFESSIONAL STANDARDS REVIEW ORGANIZATIONS (PSROs) PROGRAMS

The U.S. Congress amended the Social Security Act in 1972, establishing the PSROs to review services and items reimbursed through Medicare. Specifically, the PSROs had three responsibilities: 1) assure the quality of services; 2) respond to beneficiary complaints; and 3) protect the Medicare trust funds from fraud and abuse (Jencks, 2004). The PSROs were physician-run organizations with authority to grant or deny payments for Medicare and Medicaid services; some PSROs were funded through grants, others were financed via cooperative agreements, and some directly contracted with the federal government (Bhatia et al., 2000). Regardless of their funding and governance structures, the PSROs typically engaged in retrospective utilization review, auditing medical records and charts to ensure that Medicare and Medicaid patients received care that met recognized standards. Even though by 1981 PSROs were established in 187 of the 195 designated regions of the United States, they often were perceived as focused primarily on denying payments and restricting medical practice and were resisted by the American Medical Association, state medical societies, and many state government agencies (Luce, Bindman, & Lee, 1994). The localized structure of the PSROs, the differing funding and governance arrangements for the PSROs, and the resulting wide variations in care standards and their evaluation undoubtedly contributed to medical providers' disdain for this program (Bhatia et al., 2000).

PEER REVIEW ORGANIZATION (PRO) PROGRAM

At the same time that the PSRO program was floundering, Congress was deeply concerned about containing the inflationary costs of Medicare while sustaining enrollees' access to quality services. The PSROs were dissolved by the Peer Review Improvement Act of 1982, to be replaced by the utilization and quality control peer review organization (PRO) program. The urgency to establish PROs was further propelled by the Deficit Reduction Act of 1984, which mandated Medicare to establish and implement a prospective payment system (PPS). PPS represented a radical change in the way Medicare reimbursed hospitals for patient care, replacing service fees based on reasonable or prevailing charges with fixed fees for each case involving a patient, from admission through discharge (Luce et al., 1994). The fee paid per case by PPS depended on the resources needed for treating patients within various diagnosis-related groups (DRGs). PPS provided clear incentives for hospitals to reduce the length of stay for patients or the kinds and amounts of services provided to patients (Bhatia et al., 2000). This change in funding and incentives also gradually changed the focus of quality review organizations from primarily seeking to reduce overuse to seeking to improve the overall quality of health services.

Hence, beginning in 1984, HCFA requested proposals to contract with PROs for utilization and quality control across 54 regions in the United States and its territories (later reduced to 53 regions). During the first three contract periods (1984–1986; 1986–1989; 1989–1993) the PROs engaged mostly in retrospective utilization reviews (Bhatia et al., 2000). Specifically, the PROs were responsible for reviewing a random group of patients, assessing their DRG classifications, reviewing readmissions, reducing unnecessary hospital admissions and operations, and lowering death and complication rates. These reviews used six generic screens: 1) adequacy of discharge planning; 2) medical stability at discharge; 3) unexpected deaths; 4) nosocomial infections; 5) unscheduled returns to surgery; and 6) trauma suffered in the hospital (Luce et al., 1994).

QUALITY IMPROVEMENT ORGANIZATION (QIO) PROGRAM

By the late 1980s, the value of retrospective case reviews and traditional QA were being questioned both within the healthcare industry and by policy makers. At the request of Congress, HCFA sponsored a study by the Institute of Medicine on quality assurance for Medicare (Lohr, 1990b). The IOM study concluded that many health services did not meet standards and that retrospective case review was an unreliable method for judging the quality of services. The IOM report recommended a major shift in QA strategy toward quality improvement, urging both the PROs and JCAHO to assess clinical outcomes (Lohr, 1990a).

To address these concerns, HCFA began engaging in several quality improvement initiatives during the early 1990s. These initiatives focused on a small number of explicit, evidence-based measures of quality for inpatient care. At the same time that HCFA was piloting quality improvement initiatives with PROs, it gradually expanded the range of partners, from hospitals and physician offices to nursing homes and home health agencies (Bhatia et al., 2000). These changes in the PROs scope, intent, and activities have transformed the PRO from a confrontational agency primarily engaging in retrospective utilization review to a cooperative agency engaging in quality improvement with a wide variety of healthcare organizations (Bradley et al., 2005; Hertz & Fabrizio, 2005; "Quality Directors Give QIOs High Marks in New Study," 2005). As a result, a new designation was coined for the PROs by the newly renamed Centers for Medicare and Medicaid Services (CMS): the organizations are now called Quality Improvement Organizations (QIOs).

As the preceding discussion illustrates, both the Joint Commission and the QIOs have moved from primarily engaging in quality assurance to partnering with all forms of health service delivery organizations. Indeed, both the Joint Commission and the QIOs now champion continuous quality improvement (CQI) efforts. The next section defines and provides multiple examples of CQI principles.

CONTINUOUS QUALITY IMPROVEMENT

During the 1970s, oil shortages compelled many people in the United States to purchase fuel efficient and inexpensive cars. Although U.S. automobile manufacturers tried to produce such cars, only the Japanese were manufacturing fuel efficient yet inexpensive automobiles that were reliable and durable. The quality of these small Japanese vehicles greatly surpassed those manufactured in the United States. Newspapers, magazines, and television news asked the question, "Can America Compete with Japan?" This rapid shift in the marketplace created a new awareness among U.S. industrial leaders that quality mattered.

To address the quality deficit, automobile and other manufacturers in the United States sought the help of quality improvement experts. The contributions assured that total quality management (TQM)—referred to as continuous quality improvement (CQI) in health care—became the new paradigm for quality improvement within the United States during the 1980s and 1990s. These quality gurus and advocates included Walter A. Shewhart, W. Edwards Deming, Joseph M. Juran, and Malcolm Baldrige. They shared a common interest in improving the quality of production in manufacturing and other industries, and their extraordinary lives were intertwined both by industry experience and interest.

During the mid-1920s, Walter A. Shewhart, a physicist at Bell Laboratories, was asked to study the variations in Western Electric's production processes and formulate a means to assure that products met specifications. Rather than inspecting each product for defects, Shewhart's practical perspective led him to try to control the source of quality variation in the production process. This led him to differentiate between "common cause" and "special cause" variations. He knew that "common cause" variations in the production process—due to natural variations in raw materials, minor electrical voltage fluctuations, etc.—often were impractical to control. However, "special cause" variations—due to operator behaviors, incorrectly calibrated machinery, the substituting of different types of raw materials, etc.—could be controlled (Kolesar, 1993). His book, *Economic Control of Quality of Manufactured Product* (Shewhart, 1931), articulated these principles of statistical process control (SPC) for reducing quality variation in production processes. With editorial assistance from his protégé, W. Edwards Deming, Shewhart also wrote a monograph on quality control, *Statistical Method from the Viewpoint of Quality Control*, which introduced the Plan-Do-Check-Act (PDCA) cycle model for improving production processes (Shewhart, 1939).

Known also as the Shewhart cycle in the United States, the PDCA cycle was popularized by W. Edward Deming and it is called the Deming cycle in Japan. A statistician, Deming further developed the principles underlying TQM/CQI while working with the Japanese to reconstruct their industries after World War II. His approach with the Japanese was to help them fundamentally change work processes. Deming developed a management philosophy that encouraged worker participation in process change, focused on data-based decision making, and embraced a standardized approach to quality improvement. This management philosophy was eventually codified into 14 points (see Table 2-1).

Joseph M. Juran was a contemporary and colleague of Deming's. Born in Braila, Romania in 1904, Juran immigrated to the United States with his family in 1912, and began working at the age of 9. He earned a bachelors degree in engineering, but also excelled in mathematics and statistics.

TABLE 2-1 Deming's 14 Points

1. Create and publish to all employees a statement of the aims and purpose of the company or organization. The management must demonstrate constantly their commitment to this statement.
2. Learn the new philosophy, top management and everybody.
3. Understand the purpose of inspection, for improvement of processes and reduction of cost.
4. End the practice of awarding business on the basis of price tag alone.
5. Improve constantly and forever the system of production and service.
6. Institute training.
7. Teach and institute leadership.
8. Drive out fear. Create trust. Create a climate of innovation.
9. Optimize toward the aims and purposes of the company the efforts of teams, groups, and staff areas.
10. Eliminate exhortation for the workforce.
11a. Eliminate numerical quotas for production. Instead, learn and institute methods for improvement.
11b. Eliminate management by objective. Instead, learn the capabilities of processes and how to improve them.
12. Remove barriers that rob people of pride of workmanship.
13. Encourage education and self-improvement for everyone.
14. Take action to accomplish this transformation.

Upon graduating, he was hired as an engineer at Western Electric's Hawthorne Works in 1925. He was one of the first engineers trained by Shewhart to apply the principles of SPC. While at Western Electric, Juran championed the Pareto principle from economics, focusing attention and resources on those important quality problems that are attributable to a small number of factors (e.g., the 80/20 rule). During WWII, Juran worked as assistant to the administrator of the Foreign Economic Administration under the Office for Emergency Management. In this role, he oversaw the logistics for providing materials and supplies to allied governments and troops on both fronts. Building on this experience, another of Juran's important contributions was the "Juran Trilogy" of quality planning, quality control, and quality improvement. All of these notions were first codified in the 1951 publication of the *Quality Control Handbook* (Juran, Gryna, & Bingham, 1974); his work now is carried on by the Juran Institute (see http://www.juran.com/).

Malcolm Baldrige, Secretary of Commerce under President Reagan, died in office as a result of a rodeo accident on July 25, 1987. "Mac" Baldrige was born in Nebraska. During the course of his life he worked as a ranch hand; was a professional team roper on the rodeo circuit; served in combat during WWII as an infantry captain in the Pacific; graduated from Yale University; worked as a foundry hand in an iron company, eventually becoming its president; and was the chairman and CEO of Scovill, Inc. before serving as commerce secretary. A strong advocate of free trade and a proponent of efficiency and effectiveness in government, Baldrige is credited with transforming Scovill from a financially-troubled brass mill to a successful manufacturer of consumer products, housing, and other goods (see http://www.quality.nist.gov/Biography.htm). In his honor, the Malcolm Baldrige National Quality Award was created in 1988 for companies that display excellent performance across seven dimensions. These dimensions of quality have been continually refined and expanded from their original manufacturing base to include healthcare organizations. The Baldrige Award models excellence using a structure-process-outcomes framework.

THE CONCEPT OF CQI IN HEALTH CARE

Now that we have discussed some of the important contributors to continuous quality improvement, let's examine the concept and application of CQI in health care. The concept of continuous quality improvement can be defined as an organizational process, in which employee teams identify and address problems in their work processes. When applied across the organization, CQI creates a continuous flow of process improvements that meet or exceed customer—or patient—expectations. Inherent within this definition are five dimensions of CQI: 1) process focus, 2) customer focus, 3) data-based decision making, 4) employee empowerment, 5) organization-wide scope.

CQI focuses on the process part of Donabedian's quality conception as key to developing high quality health care. Specifically, CQI promotes the view that understanding and addressing the factors that create variation in an administrative or clinical process (e.g., long wait times, high rehospitalization rates) will produce superior patient care quality and organizational performance. Further, quality improvement should not be a one-time activity; rather it should be a normal activity, resulting in a continual flow of improvements.

Underpinning this approach are the concepts and tools of statistical process control (SPC), which Shewhart developed. For example, a manager of an ambulatory clinic has tracked an increase in complaints about patient wait time from quarterly patient satisfaction surveys. For the next month, the wait time for each patient is collected and the daily average is graphed. At the same time, data is collected about why waiting time increases, and the clinic manager finds that the "special cause" variation is driven by 1) the number of medically complex, time-consuming patients each day; 2) the training needs of a new LPN and receptionist; and 3) the over scheduling of new patients. Armed with these findings, the manager is able to work with the clinical and administrative staff to address these concerns to reduce both the variability and the average wait time.

The second element in CQI is the focus on the customer. The organization must make every effort to "delight the customer." CQI defines "customer" in broad terms. Normally, patients are thought of as the main customers in health care. CQI's view is that any person or organization that is on the downstream end of a process is a customer. For example, a doctor ordering a MRI can be considered a customer because she receives the service of the radiology department. Thus, CQI takes the position that each process has a variety of both internal and external customers. The customer focus is best exemplified in the widespread use of patient satisfaction surveys by hospitals and physician groups.

The third element in CQI is an emphasis on using data to make all quality improvement decisions. The foundation of SPC, as discussed earlier, rests on the collection, analysis, and use of data to improve processes and monitor the success of process interventions. The use of carefully collected data reduces both uncertainty and the dependence on uninformed impressions or biases for improving an organizational process. It also provides good evidence to convince skeptics that a process problem exists. Returning to our earlier example, the collected data on waiting times enabled not only the clinic manager to understand the "special cause" factors that were creating them, but also helped physicians, nurses, and front desk and other staff understand the sources of the problem.

The fourth element of CQI is employee empowerment. This empowerment is manifested by the widespread use of quality improvement teams. The typical CQI team will consist of hourly employees whose day-to-day work gives them a unique perspective and detailed knowledge of patient care processes. Another important individual for a CQI team is the facilitator, who typically provides training on CQI tools and philosophy. Members of the CQI team are not only empowered to improve their work environment, but can also become an advocate for change, overcoming resistance among other employees. In our prior example, the clinic manager worked with both clinical employees (e.g., RNs, LPNs, and the nurse supervisor) and administrative employees (e.g., receptionists, admission and billing clerks, and their supervisor) to decrease the wait times and improve patients' satisfaction with the clinic.

The final element in CQI is its strategic use across the organization, accomplished through the coordinated and continuous improvement of various operational processes. Such coordination requires a broader management philosophy for improving the organization, similar in scope and intent to the system improvement notions discussed later in this chapter. Specifically, for CQI to be effective at the organization level, three elements must be in place: executive leadership, a strategic orientation, and a commitment to cultural change.

The first element is executive leadership. Without the support of the top managers, any attempt to apply CQI principles across the healthcare organization will be likely to fail. Overcoming organizational inertia, the natural resistance to change among departmental managers and work-unit supervisors, requires an overarching organizational commitment to CQI. The second element is a strategic orientation. CQI principles must be incorporated into the strategic plans and goals of the healthcare organization. If CQI is not a budget item with clear goals that are aligned with the strategic direction of the organization, organization-wide CQI initiatives are doomed to fail. The final element is cultural change. CQI emphasizes a culture in which quality is a central value shared across the entire organization and permeating all organizational and individual activities.

APPLYING CQI

In order to make specific quality improvements, the Shewhart/Deming cycle of PDCA is generally used in manufacturing and other industries. However, during the early 1980s, the Hospital Corporation of American (HCA) modified the PDCA cycle to create the FOCUS-PDCA framework, which has become the most commonly used quality improvement framework in the healthcare industry. FOCUS stands for Find, Organize, Clarify, Understand, and Select. The addition of FOCUS clarifies the steps that need to be done prior to the implementation of any process change. The changes in the process will then be guided by the PDCA cycle.

Find means simply to find a process to improve. Problems may be identified by employees, managers, or customers. Problem identification may be helped by brainstorming about the performance problems facing a work unit or department. Once this list is complete, the next step is selecting the problem on which to focus. Problems that cause "high pain" should be chosen. Keep in mind that CQI projects are time and personnel intensive. In order to be worthwhile and be approved by management, some statement about return on investment is necessary.

Organize means to organize a team. A good CQI team has three elements. First, the team is composed of people directly involved in the process. This ensures that team members will have intimate knowledge of the process to be improved. It also has the side benefit of reducing resistance to change. Second, the team must represent the range of professional and occupational groups involved in a process. If certain stakeholders are left out of a CQI project, then the knowledge base of the project is incomplete. Moreover, any solutions developed may be resisted by those stakeholders not represented on the team. The final element is the presence of a resource person who is responsible for providing necessary CQI training and facilitating the group's activities. Without this person, the team is very likely to be ill-prepared and fail to accomplish its mandate.

Clarify is commonly done by flowcharting the process. Once a team is organized and trained, then it must turn to clarifying the process. Flowcharting documents the sequence of activities that take place in a process. Creating a usable flowchart often takes a number of meetings, particularly if there is substantial variation in how the process is performed, which may have been the reason it was selected in the first place. Flowcharting also raises the issue about the scope of the project. It is at this point that teams need to assess if the scope of their project is too big or too small.

Understand is a three-part process of identifying measures, collecting data, and analyzing it. Once there is a usable flowchart, then the team can turn to understanding the process. The first part is identifying existing or developing new quality measures; the second is collecting the data, which provide insight about how well the process is performed. Sometimes quality measures are already collected and they just need to be accessed (e.g., manual medical chart audits, patient satisfaction scores). Other times, measures need to be developed and data collected (e.g., wait times). In either case, it is important that the methods and measures used to collect data are valid and reliable. Once data has been collected, the third step, analysis, can take place. Analysis involves documenting the variation as measured and uncovering the causes of the variation. As discussed in more detail later, a wide variety of tools for uncovering causes of process variation can be used.

Select is determining the quality improvement process to implement. After the process is mapped and the process problem and its causes understood, a process improvement plan can be selected. Studying the key causes of the problem uncovered in the analysis should inspire a number of alternative plans for improving the process. The team should develop criteria for deciding which plan to use. Such criteria might involve time, costs, feasibility, and potential for employee, managerial, or customer resistance. After each alternative is weighed on the criteria, the team should be able to make a rational selection of an improvement plan.

After the selection of the quality improvement plan, the CQI team moves to the PDCA cycle. This transition is important because PDCA represents a cyclical set of actions that take place until a process improvement is deemed to have met its goals. **Planning** converts the idea proposed for process improvement into a specific set of actions. During this planning, the questions of who, what, and how should be addressed. The "Who?" question pertains to that specific group or people who will pilot test the process improvement. The "What?" question asks about the specific actions of the planned intervention, and the "How?" question addresses the step-by-step operations for implementing the intervention. Another important question is that of measurement. During the understanding part of the framework, at least one, and preferably several, measures are identified and used. In the planning stage, goals for each measure need to be developed. Often these are derived from benchmarks, which may also be used during the **Understand** part of the FOCUS-PDCA framework. The "How?" question is answered by developing a detailed set of actions to be taken in reworking and improving the process.

Once the plan is complete, then it needs to be implemented. During this stage, data are collected and implementation issues are resolved. After a suitable pilot period, the data are compared with the goals to determine if the effort is successful. Also, this is where lessons on implementation and insights into the teams' own functioning may be discussed.

The final stage of the cycle is the **A** for **Act** to hold the gains. If the goals are not met, the cycle returns to the plan step and a new process improvement idea is selected. Alternatively, if the goals are met, then the cycle terminates. However, important work often needs to be done to make sure that the improvement becomes permanent. If the improvement was pilot tested in one group (e.g., a nursing ward within a hospital), then it might be spread to other wards. Among the activities that need to be done are training personnel in the new process, revising policies, automating data collection, and educating stakeholders to reduce resistance to change.

OTHER LEADING QUALITY IMPROVEMENT MODELS

In addition to the methods discussed under CQI, there are three additional methods of quality improvement that bear brief mention, including **Six Sigma**, **reengineering**, and **ISO 9000**.

Six Sigma

Six Sigma is an extension of Joseph Juran's approach to quality improvement, and was developed by Motorola and popularized by Jack Welch at General Electric. It has been defined as a "Data-driven quality methodology that seeks to eliminate variation from a process" (Scalise, 2001). Six

Sigma employs a structured process called **DMAIC**, which stands for *Define, Measure, Analyze, Improve,* and *Control.* **Define** includes delimiting the scope of work, determining due dates, and mapping the future state of the process, including improvements. **Measure** encompasses both the creation of measures or metrics, as well as their application to determine how well a process is performing. **Analyze** further breaks down the understanding of the process, and often includes flowcharting the process. **Improve** specifies the steps that will be taken to meet the goals outlined during the define step. **Control** is about ensuring that the improvements are permanent rather than temporary.

While DMAIC guides the actual improvement project, Six Sigma also features major training and human resource components. Because of these components, many large hospital and health systems have begun adopting Six Sigma as a way to change the organization and establish a culture of quality. Such change begins with a CEO who supports the method; without top level management support, efforts like this generally founder. A champion is a senior executive (generally VP level or above) who has full-time responsibility for quality improvement efforts. Further into the organization are three levels of "belts." At the top are Master Black Belts, full-time employees who provide technical leadership and training to those running QI projects. Black Belts direct multiple projects, and Green Belts are those who lead specific projects.

Business Process Reengineering

Reengineering is another quality improvement method that has gained favor in recent years. It was popularized by the book, *Reengineering the Corporation* (Hammer & Champy, 1993). Its development was born from managers' frustration with the slow pace of other quality improvement methods. Specifically, it advocates the "radical redesign of business processes for dramatic improvement." Rather then improving existing processes, it relies on a clean sheet approach to quality improvement. It focuses on the complete end-to-end set of activities that provide value for customers. This approach has great value when it is used to rapidly pilot change within an organization and to create business options (Lillrank & Holopainen, 1998). On one hand, experience has demonstrated that large scale reengineering projects have a high risk of failure, largely because of the resistance to radical change within most organizations ("The Trouble with Re-engineering," 1995). On the other hand, large public sector health organizations, such as the Veterans Health Administration in the United States (Jha, Perlin, Kizer, & Dudley, 2003), have achieved remarkable results through reengineering. And its use is supported by the National Health System in the United Kingdom (McAdam & Corrigan, 2001).

ISO 9000

The International Organization for Standardization (ISO) is a not-for-profit organization, which provides a framework for developing voluntary technical and management system standards for international business. ISO unites a network of national standards institutes in 156 countries (see http://www.iso.org/iso/en/aboutiso/introduction/index.html). ISO's goal is to provide a world-wide consensus for the standardization of processes and services for all industries, thus benefiting consumers, businesses, and governments. ISO 9000 was proposed in 1987 and improved in 1994 to provide a non-prescriptive management system quality standard for non-technical business functions. Similar to Deming's TQM principles, ISO 9000 certification is grounded on eight principles (http://www.iso.org/iso/en/iso9000-14000/understand/qmp.html): 1) customer focus, 2) leadership, 3) involvement of people, 4) process approach, 5) system approach to management, 6) continual improvement, 7) factual approach to decision making, and 8) mutually beneficial supplier relationships. Healthcare organizations seeking ISO 9000 certification pursue the International Workshop Agreement 1:2005 standards for quality management systems, which provide guidelines for process improvements in health services (http://www.iso.ch/iso/en/CatalogueDetailPage.Catalogue Detail?CSNUMBER=41768&ICS1=11&ICS2=20&ICS3=&scopelist CATALOGUE). The healthcare organizations then demonstrate that their quality management processes meet international standards through a quality audit conducted by various ISO 9000 certification bodies.

KEY QUALITY IMPROVEMENT CONCEPTS

Across the many ways of thinking about quality and ways to improve quality, there is a common set of four key concepts: measurement, process variation, statistical process control, and quality improvement tools.

Measurement

The most basic concept in quality improvement is that of measurement and the metrics associated with it. **Measurement** is the translation of observable events into quantitative terms, while metrics are the means actually used to record phenomenon. All quality improvement efforts require numerical data because "you can't manage what you can't measure." In this way, quality improvement is driven by data-based evidence rather than subjective judgments or opinions.

Good measurement begins with the rigorous definition of the concept to be measured. It then requires the use of a measurement methodology that yields **reliable** (i.e., consistent) and **valid** (i.e., accurate) measures of the concept. Rigorous definition means that the concept to be measured (e.g., wait times) needs to be defined in very specific terms. This definition should be written and include the unit of measure. For example, wait times could be defined as the time interval between the arrival of a patient at the office and the time they are first seen by the doctor. The unit of measure is time, but the start and end points are important for assessing the reliability and validity of the measure.

Once a good definition of the concept is developed, one challenge is to measure it reliably. If every recorded wait time starts with the arrival of the patient and ends with the patient's first encounter with the doctor, then the measure should be consistent, or reliable. **Measure reliability** means that if a measure is taken at several points over time or by various people, that the measure will generally be consistent (that is, not vary too much). For example, if a person takes his/her temperature each morning, it should be close to 98.6°F each time assuming that she or he is not ill. If it substantially deviates from that temperature, then that person is either ill or the thermometer is broken and not giving consistent readings. Another example of reliability is that of reliability among people. If two nurses in a practice are measuring wait times but use different definitions of waiting, then their measurement of waiting time will not be consistent (e.g., reliable) because the two nurses are measuring the same concept, but in different ways.

Another challenge is to ensure that the measure of the concept is valid. Its validity depends on the accuracy of the measure. If two nurses use the same stopwatch to record waiting times, so long as the clock itself is accurate and the nurses adhere to the same definition of waiting, the wait times should be accurate. In other words, **validity** is the extent to which the measure used actually measures the concept. As with reliability, having a rigorous definition and method of data collection will yield a valid measure.

Process Variation and Statistical Process Control (SPC)

Process variation is the range of values that some quality metric can take as a result of different causes within the process. As Shewhart noted, these causes can take two forms: **special** and **common cause variation** (Shewhart, 1931). **Special cause variation** is due to unusual, infrequent, or unique events that cause the quality metric to deviate from its average by a statistically significant degree. **Common cause variation** is due to the usual or natural causes of variation within a process. Following Shewhart, quality improvement now involves 1) detecting and eliminating special cause variation in a process; and 2) detecting and reducing, whenever feasible, common cause variation within a process.

Statistical Process Control (SPC) is a method by which process variation is measured, tracked, and controlled with the goal of improving the quality of the process. SPC is a branch of statistics that involves time series analysis with graphic data display. The advantage of this method is that it often yields insight into the data in a way that is intuitive for most decision makers. In essence, it relies on the notion that "a picture is worth a thousand words" for its import. Quality data from a particular process are graphed across time. At some point when there is enough data, a mean and standard deviation for the data are calculated and a control chart constructed. The construction begins with the graphing of data across time. It continues with the calculation of upper and lower control limits. Think of these limits as similar to the tolerances for machined parts. Complex machinery, like aircraft, requires parts that are manufactured to very tight tolerances so that they will fit together well. The larger the tolerance, the greater the likelihood that a part will not fit the way it is supposed to fit. These limits show the range of variation where the process is thought to be "in control." Typically these limits are set at plus and minus three standard deviations. With these control limits in place, the data can be interpreted and times when the process was "out of control" investigated and remedied.

QUALITY IMPROVEMENT TOOLS

In addition to the use of control charts, there are a number of other tools that are commonly used in quality improvement activities. They can be divided into three categories: data collection, process mapping, and process analysis.

Data Collection Tools

The check sheet is a simple data collection form in which the occurrence of some event or behavior is tallied. At the end of the data collection period, they are added up. The best check sheets are those that are simple and have well-defined categories of what constitutes a particular event or behavior. For example, a doctor's office staff wanted to find out the reasons why patients showed up late. They brainstormed about the reasons and after carefully defining each reason, they developed a check sheet. The check sheet was pilot tested, and several new reasons were added while other reasons were refined. The check sheet was then employed during a month-long data collection period. They found that transportation problems and babysitting problems jointly accounted for 63% of the late shows.

Another example is the use of chart abstractions or chart audits. In this process, a check sheet is used to collect information from a patient's medical record. Most of the time this is a manual process that involves an individual looking at the medical record, finding the requested information, and recording it on a check sheet. The use of electronic medical records may take some or all of the labor out of this process, as pertinent medical information can be collected more easily or, better yet, a complete report produced at the click of a mouse.

Geographic mapping is a pictorial check sheet in which an event or problem is plotted on a map. This is often used in epidemiological studies to plot where victims of certain diseases live, work, play, etc. For example, a public health agency was trying to isolate and contain an outbreak of a virulent form of influenza. The agency plotted the places where the infected individuals' lived, worked, and/or went to school. Using that plot, they were able to focus their efforts on a specific area where the disease occurred most often.

A more focused application of geographic mapping is the workflow diagram. Simply put, this reflects the movements of people, materials, documents, or information in a process. Plotting these movements on the floor plan of a building or around a paper document can present a very vivid picture of the inefficiency of a process. With the advancement of information technology, increasingly sophisticated geographic mapping and tracking programs have become available, making this complex task easier to do.

Mapping Processes

Flowcharting is the main way that processes are mapped. A flowchart is nothing more than a picture of the sequence of steps in a process. Different actions within a process are denoted by different geometric shapes. A basic flowchart just outlines the major steps in a process. A detailed flowchart is often more useful in quality improvement. Developing such a flowchart requires substantial investigation of each aspect of the process to be charted. Determining the appropriate level of detail should be driven by the flowchart's use within the quality improvement process. A top down flowchart is often used for providing an overview of large or complex processes. It shows the major steps in the process and lists below each major step the sub-steps. The development flowchart adds another dimension to the flowchart. Often it is useful for tracking the flow of information between people. That is, the development flowchart shows the steps of the process carried out by each person, unit, or group involved in a process. Since hand-offs are often where errors may occur, this flowchart provides a target for data collection efforts.

Analyzing Processes

The cause-and-effect diagram helps to identify and organize the possible cause for a problem in a structured format. It is commonly referred to as a **fishbone diagram** for its resemblance to a fish. It is also called an **Ishikawa diagram**, in honor of Kaoru Ishikawa who developed it. The diagram begins with the problem under investigation described in a box at the right of the diagram. The fish's spine is represented by a long arrow pointing to the box. The major possible causes of the problem are arrayed as large ribs along the spine. These are broad categories of causes to which smaller ribs are attached that identify more specific causes of the problem.

A **Pareto chart** is a simple frequency chart. The frequency of each problem, reason, etc. is listed on the X-axis and the number or percent of occurrences is listed on the Y-axis. This analysis is most useful in identifying the major problems in a process and their frequency of occurrence. Another version of the frequency chart is the **histogram**, which shows the range and frequency of values for a measure. When complete, it shows the complete distribution of some variable. This is often useful in basic data analysis.

As mentioned earlier, CQI has its greatest impact if it becomes a part of the strategic mission of a healthcare organization. When that occurs, it is then possible to look beyond the boundaries of the organization and to consider ways in which the healthcare system at the local, regional, and national levels could be improved. The next section addresses why system improvement is important and outlines some of the initiatives within the United States for improving the healthcare system

SYSTEM THINKING AND HEALTHCARE QUALITY IMPROVEMENT

Within the healthcare industry, the paradigmatic shift between CQI and system improvement became fully visible with the publication of the 1999 IOM report, *To Err is Human*. Most important to the evolution of thinking about system improvement was the 2001 report, *Crossing the Quality Chasm*, which laid out an agenda for the creation of a 21st century healthcare system in the United States. The report identified six aims for health care, specifying that it should be:

- Safe—avoiding injuries to patients from care that is intended to help them;
- Effective—providing services based on scientific knowledge to all who could benefit and refraining from providing services to those not likely to benefit (e.g., avoidance of overuse and underuse);
- Patient-Centered—providing care that is respectful of and responsive to individual patient preferences, needs, and values and ensuring that patient values guide all clinical decisions;
- Timely—reducing waits and sometimes harmful delays for both those who receive and those who give care;
- Efficient—avoiding waste, including use of equipment, supplies, ideas, and energy; and,
- Equitable—providing care that does not vary in quality because of personal characteristics such as gender, ethnicity, geographic location, and socioeconomic status (IOM, 2001)

System Thinking and Active vs. Latent Errors

Taken together, the two IOM reports introduced both to the public and to many healthcare professionals a new way of thinking about quality, namely system thinking. Specifically, the authors of the IOM reports viewed many medical errors as latent and occurring in complex, tightly-linked organizations. **Latent errors** are those types of errors "whose adverse consequences may lie dormant within the system for a long time, only becoming evident when they combine with other factors to break the system's defenses" (Reason, 1990). They are likely to be spawned by "those whose activities are removed in both time and space from the direct control interface." The effects of **active errors**, on the other hand, are likely to be felt immediately and are likely to be committed by service providers directly interacting with the patient. Note that active errors are also the types of errors that are typically the ones detected by QA.

For example, consider an operating room nurse faced with setting up three different infusion pumps for the administration of anesthesia, as well as an oxygen pump. For the anesthesia to be administered without error, each pump must be set up correctly. Active errors could include overdosing the patient with an anesthetic or providing too little oxygen during surgery, either of which would potentially produce deadly harm to the patient. One potential latent error lies in having three different types of infusion pumps, each with their own set up procedure, and often with strikingly different means for turning on and off critical valves. Or the infusion pumps may have similar valves, but these may be different from those used for the oxygen pump. Moreover, dosages for different medications administered through the infusion pumps may be confused with one another, introducing other latent errors. Lastly, another latent error may be inadequate or incomplete training for the OR nurses on how to set up and operate the three different types of infusion pumps in conjunction with the oxygen.

While QA techniques probably would detect this latter problem and address it, all the other latent errors would most likely not be detected and appropriately addressed. However, we know CQI techniques are capable of detecting the other latent errors and helping to produce solutions to eliminate them. The system improvement perspective takes the knowledge gained from both QA and CQI in this example; moreover, it would focus both on (a) enabling all other hospital operating rooms to detect these latent errors and (b) diffusing the best practices for eliminating these errors.

System Interactiveness and Coupling

Beyond active and latent errors, two other important concepts are system **interactiveness** and **coupling**, which are discussed in Normal Accident Theory (Perrow, 1984).

System Interactiveness

Interactiveness is the level and type of interaction among system components; such interactions can be characterized as either linear or complex. Linear interactions follow a sequential logic: *A* interacts with *B* to produce *C*; *C* interacts with *D* to produce *E*; and so forth. Complex interactions, on the other hand, have "branching paths, feedback loops, jumps from one linear sequence to another because of proximity. The connections are not only adjacent, serial ones, but can multiply as other parts of units or subsystems are reached." Think for a moment about the following example: *A* interacts with *B* and *C* to produce *D*; *E* interacts with *A*, *C*, and *D* to produce *F*; while *G* and *E* interact with *F* to produce *H*. Now use the following to make this abstract formula more concrete: A = patient; B = admissions staff; C = nurse; D = medical complaint/history; E = attending physician; F = medical exam; G = consulting physician; H = diagnosis. As this example illustrates, even a routine visit to a family doctor often involves complex interactions. For many patients, however, obtaining a diagnosis is only the first part of an increasingly complex journey through the health system.

System Coupling

Coupling is the amount of time, distance, or slack between two elements in a system. Loosely coupled systems have more time or slack between system elements than a tightly coupled system. As the prior example illustrated, even a doctor's office contains a number of complex interactions. Complexity increases by several magnitudes in an acute care hospital, which is composed of many interacting sub-systems of care, often with tight coupling among several of the sub-systems. For example, a patient admitted into the emergency department typically will need laboratory tests and x-rays, each of which are produced by separate departments (subsystems) within the hospital. The patient's diagnosis and treatment by an

ER physician depends on these ancillary services not only being conducted correctly, but also being produced quickly and in conjunction with each other. In other words, the emergency department, imaging department, and laboratory are tightly coupled sub-systems.

HEALTH CARE AS HIGH HAZARD INDUSTRY

Because of the tightly coupled, complex interactions within healthcare organizations, Gaba (2000) argues that health care is a high hazard industry, like nuclear power or airlines. The likelihood of an adverse outcome (e.g., a medical error, long wait time, etc.) occurring increases both as a system gets more complex, and as the system's interactions become more tightly coupled. In a system characterized by complex interactions many latent errors may occur; add tightly coupled interactions between system elements, and it becomes difficult to detect and correct such errors. Consider the example of the patient admitted to the ER. Given an inaccurate or mislabeled test result or mislabeled or misread x-ray, the patient's diagnosis and treatment may be tragically wrong—although based on clinically correct decision making. Determining what went wrong, why it happened, and how to prevent its reoccurrence, requires more than simply optimizing performance by separately applying CQI techniques at the sub-system levels of the laboratory, the imaging department, or the emergency department. Instead, CQI techniques must be applied to the emergency care micro-system that encompasses each of the sub-systems. In other words, system thinking about quality improvement shifts the focus to the system encompassing the tightly coupled sub-systems. Again, the goals of system improvement are twofold: 1) to detect and eliminate latent errors in complex organizations by using CQI across the organization; and 2) to diffuse the best practices for doing so both within and across healthcare organizations. The various ways that system improvement in the United States are being attempted are discussed next.

APPROACHES TO SYSTEM IMPROVEMENT

System improvement moves quality from an issue of concern for a department or work unit, and makes it a concern for the entire organization, its network of partners, and the market and governmental institutions supporting the healthcare sector. Quality thus viewed is a property of the entire system of health care, which has to be addressed at four levels of increasing degrees of abstraction: the patient, the micro-system of care, the healthcare organization, and the healthcare environment (Berwick, 2002). The environment includes not only the network of healthcare organizations providing services, but also the incentives and restrictions they face from training, market, governmental, and accrediting institutions. The example of the patient admitted to the ER focuses on not only the patient, but also the micro-system of care. If we extend the example to include the patient's admission to the critical care unit in the hospital, discharge to a nursing home for rehabilitation, followed by home health care and ambulatory rehabilitation visits, it becomes clear that each healthcare organization involved has a responsibility to improve the quality of care for the patient. The most difficult aspect within not only the United States but also within other countries' health systems, is ensuring that there is continuity of care as a patient is transferred from one healthcare setting to another (Plochg & Klazinga, 2002; Schoen, Osborn, Hoynh, Doty, Zapert, Peugh, & Davis, 2005). Improving the quality of both healthcare practices and the continuity of care at the system level requires both governmental and industry-wide involvement and oversight.

Federal Government Initiatives

Since the 2001 publication of *Crossing the Quality Chasm*, there has been increasing activity to improve healthcare systems in the United States, involving not only governmental agencies, but also large employers, accrediting agencies, trade and professional organizations, and nonprofit organizations. The federal government's efforts to improve system quality are fivefold (Schoenbaum, Audet, & Davis, 2003):

1. The Agency for Healthcare Research and Quality (AHRQ; see http://www.ahrq.gov/) manages an active research program in quality of care and patient safety, including the Center for Quality Improvement and Patient Safety;

2. The National Quality Forum (NQF; see http://www.qualityforum .org/) is a public-private partnership working on improving quality performance measures;

3. The Patient Safety Task Force (see http://www.ahrq.gov/qual/task force/psfactst.htm) is a multi-agency research program on the quality of care and patient safety that links the AHRQ, the Centers for

Disease Control and Prevention, the CMS, and the Food and Drug Administration;

4. The Veterans Health Administration's (VHA) Quality Enhancement Research Initiative (see http://www.hsrd.research.va.gov/queri/) translates research findings and promotes innovations to improve systems of patient care (McQueen, Mittman, & Demakis, 2004); and,

5. Medicare's quality assurance program contracts with the Quality Improvement Organizations (QIOs), whose efforts to improve quality were previously discussed (see http://www.cms.hhs.gov/Quality ImprovementOrgs/).

Employer-Sponsored Initiatives

Large corporations have also become involved in improving health system quality, most notably through the Leapfrog Group, made up of more than 170 companies and corporations (see www.leapfroggroup.org/). Through partnerships with health insurance companies, medical associations, and nonprofit foundations, the Leapfrog Group has actively promoted the use of rewards and incentives for hospitals and physicians that provide high quality health services. Indeed, many of the current pay-for-performance projects either involve the Leapfrog Group or are modeled upon its efforts.

The National Business Coalition on Health (NBCH) is a national, not-for-profit organization; its members include about 90 business coalitions in 33 states, representing over 7,000 employers and about 34 million employees and their dependents (see http://www.nbch.org/more.cfm). As a coalition of coalitions, the NBCH helps member coalitions seek community health reform through value-based healthcare purchasing. Such purchasing is based both on measuring the quality and efficiency of providers and health plans and on creating incentives for rewarding providers who provide high-value care.

Accrediting Agency Initiatives

Both the Joint Commission (JCAHO; see http://www.jcaho.org/pms/index.htm) and the National Committee for Quality Assurance (NCQA; see http://www.ncqa.org/index.htm) are important contributors to system improvement in health care. During the late 1980s and early 1990s, the Joint Commission attempted to integrate performance measurement into the accreditation process through the **Indicator Measurement System**

(IMSystem). When it became clear that system improvement would require multi-faceted collaborations, the Joint Commission launched the ORYX® initiative in 1997. This initiative is open to multiple external measurement systems developed by the QIOs, NQF, CMS, AHRQ, and other organizations, and involves a wide range of activities with two overarching objectives: "1) the continuing expansion and coordination of nationally standardized core measurement capabilities and 2) increasing the use of measure data for quality improvement, benchmarking, accountability, decision making, accreditation, and research" (JCAHO; see http://www.jcaho.org/pms/reference+materials/future+goals+and+objectives.htm).

The NCQA originally began in the early 1990s as an accrediting agency for health maintenance organizations (HMOs). However, it soon assumed responsibility for reporting on HMO performance to employers and government agencies with the Health Plan Data and Information Set (HEDIS). Now it accredits not only HMOs but also preferred provider organizations (PPOs) and managed behavioral healthcare organizations (MBHOs); moreover, it has deeming authority for Medicare Advantage plans (Medicare Part C). Available to consumers, employers, and government agencies, NCQA's Health Plan Report Card (http://hprc.ncqa.org/menu.asp) assesses participating health plans throughout the United States, benchmarking them on such measures as access and services, the quality of the providers, and ability to maintain health, improve health, and help those with chronic illnesses.

Other Initiatives

A leading advocate of system-wide quality improvement, not only in the United States but worldwide, is the Institute for Healthcare Improvement (IHI; see www.ihi.org/IHI/). Founded by Donald M. Berwick, MD, the IHI is a nonprofit organization that provides training and resources for improving healthcare systems, as well as numerous programs to improve patient safety and care. It often partners with the Robert Wood Johnson Foundation (RWJF; see www.rwjf.org/index.jsp), a nonprofit philanthropy devoted to improving the health and health care of all Americans. The RWJ Foundation has been particularly focused on reducing ethnic and racial disparities in health and healthcare services, as well as pay-for-performance projects.

A leading advocate of pay-for-performance initiatives in the private sector, Bridges to Excellence (BTE; see http://www.bridgestoexcellence.org/

bte/index.htm) is a multi-state, multi-employer coalition developed by employers, physicians, health services researchers, and other experts. Its mission is to reward quality care that is safe, timely, effective, efficient, equitable, and patient-centered. Partners include HealthGrades, the Leapfrog Group, Medstat, Michael Pine and Associates, NBCH, NCQA, and WebMD; BTE is also supported by a grant from the RWJ Foundation.

Lastly, the Hospital Quality Alliance (HQA) was founded by the American Hospital Association (http://www.aha.org/aha/key_issues/qualityalliance/index.html), the Federation of American Hospitals (http://www.fah.org/issues/quality_initiative/), and the Association of American Medical Colleges (http://www.aamc.org/quality/hospitalalliance/start.htm). A national public-private collaboration, the HQA encourages hospitals to voluntarily collect and report hospital quality performance information. As we discuss later, the HQA makes important information about hospital performance accessible to the public, helping to inform and invigorate efforts to improve quality. CMS and the Joint Commission participate in the HQA, along with the AHA, the FAH, the AAMC, the American Medical Association, the American Nurses Association, the National Association of Children's Hospitals and Related Organizations, American Association of Retired People, the American Federation of Labor and Council of Industrial Organizations, the Consumer-Purchaser Disclosure Project, the AHRQ, the NQF, and the U.S. Chamber of Commerce.

These various initiatives have had a positive impact on improving healthcare quality in the United States and elsewhere, but much still remains to be done. A latter section in this chapter discusses the quality and performance challenges facing healthcare organizations, especially in the United States.

A good place to start when considering the quality and performance challenges facing healthcare organizations and institutions is an assessment of what has been done. To that end, the Commonwealth Fund recently published an Issue Brief entitled, *Medical Errors: Five Years after the IOM Report* (Bleich, 2005).

ASSESSING HEALTHCARE SYSTEM IMPROVEMENT

In its report, *Crossing the Quality Chasm* (Institute of Medicine, 2001), the IOM recommended a fourfold strategy for improving system quality:

1. Establish a Center for Patient Safety within the Agency for Healthcare Research and Quality (AHRQ);
2. Develop a nationwide mandatory error-reporting system for adverse events that cause death and serious harm, as well as voluntary error-reporting systems for events that cause minimal harm;
3. Raise explicit performance standards for patient safety and enforce them through licensing, certification, and accreditation; and
4. Implement safety systems and best practices at the delivery level in healthcare organizations.

As noted in the previous section, many of these recommendations are being carried out. AHRQ's Center for Quality Improvement and Patient Safety has helped address the first recommendation, as has its other efforts to support research and disseminate best practices on patient safety. Also, JCAHO and NCQA have begun fulfilling the third recommendation by requiring healthcare organizations and health plans, respectively, to meet and improve patient safety standards. Moreover, CMS, BTE, JCAHO, the Leapfrog Group, QIOs, and the IHI are collaborating to improve safety systems and disseminate best practices among healthcare organizations, helping to address the fourth recommendation.

The second recommendation, to develop mandatory and voluntary error-reporting systems, has been much harder to initiate. As of 2005, mandatory reporting was required in only 22 states (Bleich, 2005), and there is a great deal of variation in what is reported and the transparency of this reporting to the public (McQueen, Mittman, & Demakis, 2004). Moreover, there is considerable opposition to voluntary reporting systems from hospital administrators and from physicians, largely because of the threat of malpractice litigation (Andrus, Villasenor, Kettelle, Roth, Sweeney, & Matolo, 2003; Weissman, Annas, Epstein, Schneider, Clarridge, Kirle, Gotsanis, Feibelmann, & Ridley, 2005).

HEALTHCARE SYSTEM IMPROVEMENT CHALLENGES

The difficulty that the United States has encountered in implementing the IOM's error-reporting recommendation underscores not only this but also other performance and quality improvement challenges. These challenges occur not only because of legal constraints (Pawlson & O'Kane, 2004), but also because of the uncertainty in diagnosing and providing medical treatments (Lillrank & Liukko, 2004), deficits in the information technology infrastructure in the health system (Ortiz, Meyer, & Burstin, 2002; Schoenbaum et al., 2003), and the economic incentives within the healthcare financing system (McNeil, 2001). We discuss each of these four challenges to conclude this chapter.

Reforming Medical Malpractice

Medical malpractice litigation exists in part to deter carelessness (i.e., negligence) on the part of medical providers; it does so by allowing patients to be compensated for harm and suffering (Wood, 1998). The evidence for the effectiveness of medical malpractice litigation in deterring poor quality is meager. Not only does it do little to improve healthcare quality (Pawlson & O'Kane, 2004), but it also does much to decrease healthcare quality in two ways. First, the so-called defensive practice of medicine increases the overuse of unnecessary medical services, especially diagnostic tests and imaging services (Rubin & Mendelson, 1994). Both physicians and hospitals are likely to order more, rather than less, testing to avoid legal liability for a misdiagnosis or failure to provide treatment, even if the testing or treatment may have limited benefit. Second, inflated medical malpractice awards have periodically brought about crises in malpractice insurance costs. When malpractice insurance becomes unaffordable, this induces many physicians to restrict or leave the practice of medicine and contributes to the scarcity of needed medical services, such as obstetrics (Amon & Winn, 2004).

Understandably, physicians and hospitals are particularly sensitive to the disincentives that medical malpractice litigation poses for reporting medical errors. For example, without immunity from medical malpractice prosecution, physicians are reluctant to report medical errors (Andrus, Villasenor, Kettelle, Roth, Sweeney, & Matolo, 2003). Reforming medical malpractice legislation at the national level to provide immunity to physicians reporting medical errors would be one way to address this issue. Another would be to encourage medical error reporting through incentives from the companies issuing medical malpractice insurance (Pawlson & O'Kane, 2004).

Others argue that the system of malpractice litigation should be moved from the courts to third-party arbitration and that the National Practitioner Data Bank should be more transparent, to allow for data mining and quality improvement efforts (Lehrman, 2003). Still others argue that the standard of care on which malpractice is judged should be empirically determined, encouraging the use of practice guidelines and protecting physicians who follow them (Hall & Green, 2004). A more refined argument along this vein is that malpractice cases should distinguish among three categories of care: effective care, preference-sensitive care, and supply-sensitive care (Wennberg & Peters, 2004).

Effective care has established clinical evidence that it is the most beneficial treatment or diagnostic test for a particular illness. For such care, a legal standard should be that all of those in need should receive the treatment. **Preference-sensitive care**, in contrast, occurs when various treatments or tests are available for a specific illness, each with different risks and benefits. The law should adopt a standard of informed patient choice for the treatment that best advances patient preferences. Lastly, **supply-sensitive care** occurs when less intensive care can be substituted for more intensive care with essentially equivalent outcomes, and applies particularly to those with chronic illnesses. For such care, providers should be protected under the "respectable minority" doctrine if they adopt conservative patterns of practice (Wennberg & Peters, 2004).

Accounting for Medical Uncertainty

The distinctions among effective, preference-sensitive, and supply-sensitive care point to different aspects of medical uncertainty facing both providers and patients. As we have emphasized, CQI and other quality improvement approaches are effective to the extent that they reduce process variation in the provision of health care. Care processes that can be circumscribed sufficiently to be found effective—what Wennberg and his colleagues call effective care (Wennberg, 2005; Wennberg & Peters, 2004) and others label evidence-based medicine (McNeil, 2001)—have little uncertainty. Lillrank and his colleagues note that effective care assumes that standard operating procedures for a care process can be developed for (a) assessing a patient, (b) specifying decision rules for generating an appropriate treatment, and (c) implementing a treatment to eliminate or alleviate the patient's illness (Lillrank, 2002, 2003; Lillrank & Liukko, 2004). In other words, given a patient with a particular condition, specific medical personnel examine and diagnose the patient; determine the appropriate treatment based on existing knowledge and decision rules; and deploy certain facilities, equipment, and medical supplies to treat the patient and to produce an expected outcome. CQI helps to create standard operating procedures so that each aspect of the care process is repeated the same way each time a patient with a particular condition is seen. For instance, the process of examining a patient with an apparent cold, diagnosing a viral upper respiratory infection, and prescribing decongestants and antihistamines, as well as adequate fluids and rest, are steps that should and can be repeated from one patient to another without error by a primary care physician or nurse practitioner.

However, most healthcare processes are not standard. Many healthcare processes have more than one type of input and two or more types of alternative outputs. Lillrank and his colleagues (Lillrank, 2002, 2003; Lillrank & Liukko, 2004) call these *routine* types of care processes. For example, one patient with type II diabetes may have hypertension and glaucoma, while another type II diabetes patient may be obese and have impaired circulation. While the dominant disease state is the same and similar health outcomes may be sought for both patients, the treatment for each patient will differ because of their co-morbidities. With the diabetes type II patient with co-morbidity, a single standard operating procedure is not appropriate. Rather, the physician—and the patient—must make choices across different procedures for treating each of the diseases.

Hence, routine healthcare processes are more likely to encompass what Wennberg and his colleagues (Wennberg, 2005; Wennberg & Peters, 2004) call preference-sensitive care. On one hand, some obese patients may be willing and able to use both exercise and diet to control diabetes type II, if the physician can prescribe appropriate medication and devices to improve blood circulation and prevent leg cramps. On the other hand, other obese patients may seek gastric bypass surgery, while still others may seek only nutrition and dietary counseling along with support groups. Whether physicians can accommodate these different patient preferences is also influenced by supply-sensitive care. In a community with a large number of bariatric surgeons and few registered dieticians, patients face a greater likelihood that they will be asked to consider the high-risk treatment alternative of gastric bypass surgery. In contrast, if the community has a high degree of managed care penetration by health maintenance organizations (HMOs), physical therapy and dietary counseling may be the predominant services available.

Lastly, some healthcare processes are non-routine. In many such instances, the inputs provided by the patients' symptoms are unclear and not easily diagnosed (Lillrank, 2002, 2003; Lillrank & Liukko, 2004). In other instances, given a confirmed diagnosis, the efficacy of various treatments for the disease may be uncertain, with no clear understanding of the possible outcomes (McNeil, 2001). In the first case, an iterative process of testing and excluding various diseases that manifest similar symptoms is necessary. In the second case, a similar iterative process of trying various treatments is required. In both cases, physicians' interpretive and information seeking capabilities account for much of the variation in the care process. Here, especially, preference-sensitive and supply-sensitive care processes come into play. Some patients may demand highly invasive and risky diagnostic tests or treatments, while other patients prefer low risk, non-invasive testing or treatments. Moreover, some physicians may recommend invasive diagnostics and treatments rather than non-invasive tests and treatments, particularly if such tests and treatments are readily accessible. Again, patients' access to healthcare organizations and the restrictions placed on such access by their health insurance, especially in the United States, will have a great deal of influence on when and whether patients receive more or less invasive tests and treatments.

Significantly, the quality problems facing standard, routine, and non-routine healthcare processes differ as follows (Lillrank & Liukko, 2004, p. 43):

Non-compliance with a standard process produces a deviation from the target.

Inappropriate selection from known alternatives in a routine process produces an error.

Improper assessment of input [or an output] in a non-routine process produces a failure.

To address these different types of quality problems, healthcare managers and health professionals must use appropriate methods. Standard healthcare processes can see significant quality improvement through CQI and other quality system approaches. The quality of non-routine healthcare processes, in contrast, will be improved by the clinical experience and intuition of the health providers. Here, healthcare organizations benefit from a strong quality culture—developed by health professionals' clinical training and reinforced by organizational and institutional values, such as those espoused by QA proponents. Routine healthcare processes, of course, lie between these two extremes and benefit both from CQI and a

strong QA culture. Recall the difficulties healthcare providers have in ensuring that there is continuity of care as a patient is transferred from one
healthcare setting to another. On one hand, the uncertainty involved in
medical care often is reduced as patients move from primary to secondary
to tertiary care settings, as non-routine processes in physician offices become the routine, albeit, complex and tightly-coupled processes performed in diagnostic clinics, surgical centers, and hospitals. On the other
hand, the method of sharing medical or health records between healthcare
providers across these different settings often creates new quality problems.
The inadequacies of the health information technology (HIT) infrastructure linking healthcare facilities and providers are discussed next.

DEVELOPING A NATIONAL INFORMATION TECHNOLOGY INFRASTRUCTURE

Currently, most healthcare providers rely on faxing or couriering paper patient records from one healthcare setting to another. Incomplete, missing,
or poorly organized information within these health records may cause
problems ranging from duplicative diagnostic tests, to delays in diagnosis
and treatment, to adverse drug-drug interactions, to surgery on the wrong
limb or the wrong patient. "If the state of the US medical technology is
one of our great treasures, then the state of US HIT is one of our great dis-
graces" (Kleinke, 2005, p. 1247). Despite HIT investments by insurers
and large hospitals, only the two largest integrated healthcare systems in
the United States—the Veterans Health Administration and Kaiser Per-
manente, a California-based HMO—have the HIT infrastructure that allows patients' electronic health records to be accessed by providers
throughout those organizations. This situation represents a massive market failure, and has led to multiple calls for intervention by the federal government (Halvorson, 2005; Kleinke, 2005; Middleton, 2005; Shortliffe,
2005). As a result, the U.S. federal government has set a target of 2014 for
establishing a national information technology infrastructure for health care.

[S]uch a system would dramatically improve the quality of patient care and
reduce the nation's healthcare costs by:

- Making the patient's up-to-date medical record instantly available whenever
  and wherever it is needed and authorized;
- Avoiding costly duplicate tests and unnecessary hospitalizations;

- Providing health professionals with the best and latest treatment options for the patient's needs;
- Helping eliminate medical errors;
- Streamlining the reporting of public health information for early detection and response to disease outbreaks and potential bioterrorism;
- Creating opportunities to gather non-identifiable information about health outcomes for research to identify the most effective treatment options;
- Providing better, more current medical records at lower costs; and,
- Protecting privacy (HHS, 2004).

To fulfill the above goals, a national information technology infrastructure for health care must overcome certain barriers. These barriers include ensuring that (a) electronic health records (EHRs) use a shared medical terminology and standard codes; (b) different EHR systems are interoperable, allowing the sharing of information; (c) shared EHR information is secure; (d) legal barriers to collaboration on EHR systems are removed; and (e) the costs for implementing EHRs in physician offices and other small healthcare organizations are offset (Yasnoff, Humphreys, Overhage, Detmer, Brennan, Morris, Middleton, Bates, & Fanning, 2004). The latter costs occur because there is a significant EHR adoption gap between large and small healthcare organizations; a negative business case for EHRs in physician practices, small clinics, and ambulatory centers; and limited access to HIT expertise and implementation support within these settings (Bates, 2005; HHS, 2005).

To overcome these barriers, the President of the United States issued an executive order in 2004 authorizing the establishment of the Office of the National Coordinator for Health Information Technology within the Department of Health and Human Services (HHS; see http://www.white house.gov/news/releases/2004/04/20040427-4.html). The National Coordinator, David Brailer, MD, PhD, has broad responsibility to establish a national health information technology infrastructure that will inform and interconnect clinicians, personalize care, and improve the population health of the United States (http://www.hhs.gov/healthit/goals.html). As indicated in the sidebar, the Office of the National Coordinator for Health Information Technology has initiated five projects.

1. Working with the Commission on Systemic Interoperability, authorized by the 2003 Medicare Modernization Act to make recommendations for establishing a national health information technology

infrastructure; its report, *Ending the Document Game: Connecting and Transforming Your Healthcare through Information Technology*, issued in October, 2005, has 12 recommendations (http://www.hhs.gov/healthit/comsystinter.html);

2. Overseeing the Consolidated Health Informatics Initiative (CHI) to establish health information interoperability standards for sharing EHRs and other health data among all federal agencies and departments (http://www.hhs.gov/healthit/chi.html);

3. Establishing the American Health Information Community, a federally-chartered commission, tasked with making "recommendations to HHS on how to make health records digital and interoperable, and assure that the privacy and security of those records are protected" (http://www.hhs.gov/healthit/ahic.html);

4. Awarding contracts to three different public-private groups in October, 2005, for accelerating adoption of HIT (http://www.hhs.gov/news/press/2005pres/20051006a.html), and to four consortia of healthcare and HIT organizations in November, 2005, for developing prototypes for a Nationwide Health Information Network architecture (http://www.hhs.gov/news/press/2005pres/20051110.html); and,

5. Proposing regulatory changes to allow exceptions to the Stark and anti-kickback laws, thus enabling hospitals and other healthcare organizations to furnish hardware, software, and training services to physicians for interoperable e-prescribing and EHR systems (http://www.hhs.gov/healthit/e-prescribing.html).

While a fully operational national health information technology infrastructure is needed to improve the quality of health care in the United States, the widespread adoption of EHRs, e-prescribing, and other HIT also requires aligning the economic incentives between providers and payers (Poon, Jha, Christino, Honour, Fernandopulle, Middleton, Newhouse, Leape, Bates, Blumenthal, & Kaushal 2006).

Aligning Economic Incentives

One of the dilemmas facing any healthcare financing system is ensuring that payments to healthcare providers reward them for services and outcomes that improve the health of patients. In other words, healthcare providers should provide effective care for standard cases where the diagnosis or treatments are evidence-based, preference-sensitive care for other routine and non-routine cases, and minimize or eliminate supply-sensitive care. On one hand, fee-for-service financing systems are prone to overuse of services because providers induce their own demand for services (Rice & Labelle, 1989), i.e., generate supply-sensitive care (Wennberg, 2005). On the other hand, capitated financing systems, where physicians are salaried or providers are paid prospectively per patient, are prone to underuse of effective and, especially, preference-sensitive services (Blomqvist & Leger, 2005; Iversen, 2004; Lien, Ma, & McGuire, 2004).

As mentioned previously, the Leapfrog Group, Bridges to Excellence, and Medicare are experimenting with **pay-for-performance (PFP)** programs in hospitals, physician group practices, skilled nursing facilities, and home health agencies (Beich, Scanlon, Ulbrecht, Ford, & Ibrahim, 2006; Bokhour et al., 2006; Chassin, 2006; Galvin, 2006; Grossbart, 2006; Hackbarth, 2006; Levin-Scherz, DeVita, & Timbie, 2006; Nahra, Reiter, Hirth, Shermer, & Wheeler, 2006). Ideally, as an incentive program, PFP should use evidence-based performance measures to reward healthcare providers for improving both patient safety and the quality of health care, while avoiding the rationing of care services simply to reduce costs (Baumann & Dellert, 2006). The latter concern is particularly important to physicians, many of whom are skeptical and some of whom are opposed to PFP programs as yet another means to reduce physician autonomy and income (Bodenheimer, May, Berenson, & Coughlan, 2005; Steiger, 2005; Weber, 2005).

The three most notable PFP initiatives in the United States include the Leapfrog Group's Hospital Rewards Program (see https://leapfrog.medstat.com/hrp/index.asp); the Bridges to Excellence PFP programs that reward physicians who improve cardiac and diabetes care outcomes and use HIT to improve patient care (see http://www.bridgestoexcellence.org/bte/physicians/home.htm); and the federal government. Medicare is pursuing ten PFP initiatives and demonstration projects as part of its overall Quality Initiative that was launched in 2001 (CMS, 2005c; Kuhn, 2005).

1. The *Hospital Quality Initiative* is a voluntary reporting by hospitals of 20 quality measures vetted by the CMS, HQA, JCAHO, NQF

and the QIOs. There is a strong incentive for hospitals to report this information because the Medicare Modernization Act of 2003 authorizes CMS to reduce annual payments by 0.4% if the 10 quality measures are not submitted (CMS, 2005b). The results of these measures are reported in the website, *Hospital Compare* (www .hospitalcompare.hhs.gov).

2. In partnership with Premier Inc., a nationwide organization of not-for-profit hospitals, CMS launched the *Premier Hospital Quality Incentive Demonstration* in March, 2003 and announced the first year results in November, 2005 ("Pay for Performance Works Says CMS," 2006). PFP is explicit in this demonstration; CMS increases Medicare patient payments for the participating top performing hospitals (http:// new.cms.hhs.gov/HospitalQualityInits/35_HospitalPremier.asp).

3. The *Physician Group Practice Demonstration*, authorized by the Medicare, Medicaid, and SCHIP Benefits and Improvement Act of 2000, is a 3-year PFP project that targets large group practices with at least 200 physicians. It began in April, 2005 with 10 participating physician group practices located in 10 different states (CMS, 2005e). Each of the group practices will be rewarded for coordinating the care of chronically ill and high cost beneficiaries in an efficient and effective manner. The "groups will have incentives to use electronic records and other care management strategies that, based on clinical evidence and patient data, improve patient outcomes and lower total medical costs" (CMS, 2005e).

4. The *Medicare Care Management Performance Demonstration* is modeled on the Bridges to Excellence framework. It is a 3-year pay-for-performance demonstration with physicians to promote the adoption and use of HIT to improve the quality of patient care for chronically ill Medicare patients. Doctors who meet or exceed performance standards established by CMS in clinical delivery systems and patient outcomes will receive bonus payments. In contrast to the *Physician Group Practice Demonstration*, this demonstration focuses on small and medium-sized physician practices (CMS, 2005c).

5. The *Medicare Health Care Quality Demonstration* projects, authorized by Section 646 of the 2003 Medicare Modernization Act, have a 5-year mandate to encourage a variety of quality improvements, including improving patient safety, reducing variations in utilization

via evidence-based care and practice guidelines, encouraging shared decision making, and using culturally and ethnically appropriate care (CMS, 2005c). Physician groups, integrated delivery systems, and regional healthcare consortia are eligible for the 8–12 demonstration projects, with proposals due in two phases during 2006 (CMS, 2005d).

6. The *Chronic Care Improvement Program* pilot tests a population-based model of disease management. Participating organizations are paid a monthly per beneficiary fee for managing a population of chronically ill Medicare patients with advanced congestive heart failure and/or complex diabetes. Nine sites have been selected: Humana in South and Central Florida; XLHealth in Tennessee; Aetna in Illinois; LifeMasters in Oklahoma; McKesson in Mississippi; CIGNA in Georgia; Health Dialog in Pennsylvania; American Healthways in Washington, DC and Maryland; and Visiting Nurse Service of NY and United Healthcare in Queens and Brooklyn, New York (CMS, 2005c).

7. The *ESRD Disease Management Demonstration* tests the effectiveness of disease management models to increase quality of care for end stage renal disease (ESRD) patients. Five percent of the payment will be linked to ESRD-related quality measures. Three organizations are participating in this multi-state project: DaVita, Fresenius Medical Care North America, and Evercare of Georgia (CMS, 2005a).

8. The *Disease Management Demonstration for Severely Chronically Ill Medicare Beneficiaries* tests whether disease management and prescription drug coverage improves health outcomes and reduces costs for beneficiaries with illnesses such as congestive heart failure, diabetes, or coronary artery disease. Three disease management organizations are participating: XLHealth in Texas; CorSolutions in Louisiana; and HeartPartners in California and Arizona. They receive a monthly payment for every beneficiary they enroll to provide disease management services and a comprehensive drug benefit, and must guarantee that there will be a net reduction in Medicare expenditures as a result of their services (CMS, 2005c).

9. *Disease Management Demonstration for Chronically Ill Duel-Eligible Beneficiaries* focuses on dually (Medicare & Medicaid) eligible beneficiaries in Florida who suffer from advanced-stage congestive heart failure, diabetes, or coronary heart disease. The demonstration com-

bines the resources of the state's Medicaid pharmacy benefit with a disease management activity funded by Medicare to coordinate the services of both programs and achieve improved quality with lower total program costs. LifeMasters, the demonstration organization, is being paid a fixed monthly amount per beneficiary and is at risk for 100% of its fees if performance targets are not met. Savings above the targeted amount will be shared equally between CMS and LifeMasters (CMS, 2005c).

10. *Care Management for High Cost Beneficiaries* targets beneficiaries who are both high-cost and high-risk. The payment methodology will be similar to that implemented in the Chronic Care Improvement Program, with participating providers required to meet relevant clinical quality standards, as well as to guarantee savings to the Medicare program (CMS, 2005c).

While the effectiveness of PFP initiatives is still being scrutinized by health services researchers and policy makers, preliminary evidence shows some support for the effectiveness of PFP programs in hospitals and within disease management programs (Beich, Scanlon, Ulbrecht, Ford, & Ibrahim, 2006; Grossbart, 2006; Levin-Scherz, DeVita, & Timbie, 2006; Nahra, Reiter, Hirth, Shermer, & Wheeler, 2006). Experts caution that these early studies all exhibit some flaws in their research designs, are positively biased because the sample of providers volunteered to be part of the PFP programs, and that generalizing the results to other settings and to non-volunteer providers may not be warranted (Chassin, 2006; Galvin, 2006). Nonetheless, both the Medicare Payment Advisory Commission (MedPac) and CMS believe that the effectiveness of PFP programs is sufficient to ask Congress to link Medicare payments to quality (Hackbarth, 2006; "Pay For Performance Works," 2006).

CONCLUSION

Healthcare quality may be defined in various ways, with differing implications for healthcare providers, patients, third-party payers, policy makers, and other stakeholders. High quality health services are co-produced by both providers and patients. On one hand, such care should achieve the desired health outcomes for individuals, matching their preferences for various types of outcomes. On the other hand, health services should adhere to professional standards and scientific evidence, consistent with the clinical focus and preferences of healthcare providers for effectiveness. Moreover, such services should achieve desired health outcomes for populations, matching the societal preferences of policy makers and third-party payers for efficiency.

Quality is important in health care because there are limited resources to improve the health of both individuals and the population as a whole. High quality healthcare services avoid the inappropriate use of resources that occur when services are underused, overused, or misused. The overuse of health services not only increases the overall costs of care, but also exposes patients to undue risks. In contrast, the underuse of health services leads to unacceptable levels of morbidity and mortality within a population. Lastly, misuse of health services directly harms patients and wastes resources. Both ethical and economic concerns are raised by each of these quality problems. Modern attempts to guarantee healthcare quality have ranged from quality assurance to continuous quality improvement to system improvement.

The United States is engaged in multiple governmental initiatives and public-private partnerships to improve the quality of the healthcare system that include the Agency for Healthcare Research and Quality, the National Quality Forum, the Patient Safety Task Force, the VHA's Quality Enhancement Research Initiative, and the QIOs that contract with Medicare. Most employer-sponsored initiatives originate with either the Leapfrog Group or the National Business Coalition on Health; accrediting agency initiatives are associated with the Joint Commission and the National Committee for Quality Assurance. Other notable quality improvement initiatives have been produced by the Institute for Healthcare Improvement, the Robert Wood Johnson Foundation, the Bridges to Excellence coalition, and the Hospital Quality Alliance.

Taken together these efforts have addressed many of the goals for improving the quality of health care as presented in the IOM's report, *Crossing the Quality Chasm*. Nonetheless, in the United States four significant challenges remain: 1) reforming medical malpractice; 2) accounting for and reducing medical uncertainty; 3) developing a national information technology infrastructure; and 4) aligning economic incentives. Meeting these challenges will take both talent and persistence. As the next generation of healthcare managers emerges, healthcare quality and performance improvement will be important factors for judging the competencies of those managers. In other words, understanding and appropriately applying the concepts of QA, CQI, and system improvement will be essential for healthcare managers.

DISCUSSION QUESTIONS

1. Why is quality of care a concern in the United States and around the world?
2. How can quality of care be measured from a patient's perspective? A healthcare provider's perspective? A purchaser's perspective?
3. In what ways has the concern for quality of care changed in the last 150 years—from the time of Florence Nightingale to that of Donald Berwick?
4. What are the pros and cons of different methods for improving the delivery of care within the healthcare organizations?
5. What barriers do healthcare providers and organizations face when attempting to improve care?

REFERENCES

Amon, E., & Winn, H. N. (2004). Review of the professional medical liability insurance crisis: lessons from Missouri. *American Journal of Obstetrics and Gynecology, 190*(6), 1534–1538; discussion 1538–1540.

Andrus, C. H., Villasenor, E. G., Kettelle, J. B., Roth, R., Sweeney, A. M., & Matolo, N. M. (2003). "To Err Is Human": uniformly reporting medical errors and near misses, a naive, costly, and misdirected goal. *Journal of the American College of Surgery, 196*(6), 911–918.

Bates, D. W. (2005). Physicians and ambulatory electronic health records. *Health Affairs, 24*(5), 1180–1189.

Baumann, M. H., & Dellert, E. (2006). Performance measures and pay for performance. *Chest, 129*(1), 188–191.

Beich, J., Scanlon, D. P., Ulbrecht, J., Ford, E. W., & Ibrahim, I. A. (2006). The role of disease management in pay-for-performance programs for improving the care of chronically ill patients. *Medical Care Research and Review, 63*(1_suppl), 96S–116.

Berwick, D. M. (2002). A user's manual for the IOM's 'Quality Chasm' report. *Health Affairs, 21(3)*, 80–90.

Bhatia, A. J., Blackstock, S., Nelson, R., & Ng, T. S. (2000). Evolution of quality review programs for Medicare: quality assurance to quality improvement. *Health Care Financing Review, 22*(1), 69–74.

Bleich, S. (2005). *Medical errors: five years after the IOM report* (Issue Brief). New York: Commonwealth Fund.

Blomqvist, A., & Leger, P. T. (2005). Information asymmetry, insurance, and the decision to hospitalize. *Journal of Health Economics, 24*(4), 775–793.

Bodenheimer, T., May, J. H., Berenson, R. A., & Coughlan, J. (2005). Can money buy quality? Physician response to pay for performance. *Issue Brief Center for Studying Health System Change*(102), 1–4.

Bokhour, B. G., Burgess, J. F., Jr., Hook, J. M., White, B., Berlowitz, D., Guldin, M. R., et al. (2006). Incentive implementation in physician practices: a qualitative study of practice executive perspectives on pay for performance. *Medical Care Research and Review, 63*(1_suppl), 73S–95.

Bosk, C. L. (1979). *Forgive and remember: managing medical failure.* Chicago: University of Chicago Press.

Bradley, E. H., Carlson, M. D., Gallo, W. T., Scinto, J., Campbell, M. K., & Krumholz, H. M. (2005). From adversary to partner: have quality improvement organizations made the transition? *Health Services Research, 40*(2), 459–476.

Chassin, M. R. (1997). Assessing strategies for quality improvement. *Health Affairs, 16*(3), 151–161.

Chassin, M. R. (2006). Does paying for performance improve the quality of health care? *Medical Care Research and Review, 63*(1_suppl), 122S–125.

CMS. (2005a, September 15). *Details for ESRD Disease Management Demonstration.* Retrieved March 1, 2006, from http://new.cms.hhs.gov/DemoProjectsEvalRpts/MD/itemdetail.asp?filterType=none&filterByDID=-99&sortByDID=3&sortOrder=ascending&itemID=CMS024167

CMS. (2005b, December). *Hospital quality initiative: overview.* Retrieved March 1, 2006, from http://www.cms.hhs.gov/HospitalQualityInits/downloads/HospitalOverview200512.pdf

CMS. (2005c, January 31). *Medicare "pay for performance (P4P)" initiatives.* Retrieved March 1, 2006, from http://new.cms.hhs.gov/apps/media/press/release.asp?Counter=1343

CMS. (2005d). *Medicare health care quality demonstration programs fact sheet.* Retrieved March 1, 2006, from http://www.cms.hhs.gov/DemoProjectsEvalRpts/downloads/MMA646_FactSheet.pdf

CMS. (2005e, January 31). *Medicare physician group practice demonstration fact sheet.* Retrieved March 1, 2006, from http://new.cms.hhs.gov/DemoProjectsEvalRpts/downloads/PGP_Fact_Sheet.pdf

Cooper, M. R. (1999). Quality assurance and improvement. In L. F. Wolper (Ed.), *Health care administration: planning, implementing, and managing organized delivery systems (3rd ed.,* pp. 545–573). Gaithersburg, MD: Aspen Publishers, Inc.

Davis, M. (2003). What can we learn by looking for the first code of professional ethics? *Theoretical Medicine and Bioethics, 24*(5), 433–454.

Delpierre, C., Cuzin, L., Fillaux, J., Alvarez, M., Massip, P., & Lang, T. (2004). A systematic review of computer-based patient record systems and quality of care: more randomized clinical trials or a broader approach? *International Journal for Quality in Health Care, 16*(5), 407–416.

Donabedian, A. (1966). Evaluating the quality of medical care. *Milbank Memorial Fund Quarterly, 44*(3), Suppl:166–206.

Donabedian, A. (1986). Quality assurance in our health care system. *Quality Assurance, 1*(1), 6–12.

Flexner, A. (1972, c1910). *Medical education in the United States and Canada: a report to the Carnegie Foundation for the Advancement of Teaching.* New York: Arno Press.

Fonarow, G. C. (2005). Practical considerations of beta-blockade in the management of the post-myocardial infarction patient. *Am Heart J, 149*(6), 984–993.

Gaba, D. (2000). Structural and organizational issues in patient safety: A comparison of health care to other high-hazard industries. *California Management Review, 43*(1), 83–100.

Galvin, R. S. (2006). Evaluating the performance of pay for performance. *Medical Care Research and Review, 63*(1_suppl), 126S–130.

Gandhi, T. K, Weingart, S. N, Borus, J., Seger, A. C., Peterson, J., Burdick, E., et al. (2003). Adverse drug events in ambulatory care. *New England Journal of Medicine, 348*(16), 1556.

Gilpatrick, E. (1999). *Quality improvement projects in health care: problem solving in the workplace.* Thousand Oaks, CA: Sage Publications.

Gonzales, R., Steiner, J. F., & Sande, M. A. (1997). Antibiotic prescribing for adults with colds, upper respiratory tract infections and bronchitis by ambulatory care physicians. *Journal of the American Medical Association, 278*, 901–904.

Grossbart, S. R. (2006). What's the return? Assessing the effect of "pay-for-performance" initiatives on the quality of care delivery. *Medical Care Research and Review, 63*(1_suppl), 29S–48.

Hackbarth, G. (2006). Commentary. *Medical Care Research and Review, 63*(1_suppl), 117S–121.

Hall, M. A., & Green, M. D. (2004). Malpractice litigation reform: empirical approaches to establishing the legal standard of care. *Journal of Medical Practice Management, 19*(5), 279–282.

Halvorson, G. C. (2005). Wiring health care. *Health Affairs, 24*(5), 1266–1268.

Hammer, M., & Champy, J. (1993). *Reengineering the corporation: a manifesto for business revolution.* New York: Harper Business.

Henry, B., Woods, S., & Nagelkerk, J. (1990). Nightingale's perspective of nursing administration. *Nursing & Health Care, 11*(4), 201–206.

Hertz, K. T., & Fabrizio, N. (2005). The many faces of QIOs, and what their latest incarnation means for your practice. *MGMA Connexion, 5*(7), 41, 42–45.

HHS. (2004, May 6). *Harnessing information technology to improve health care.* Retrieved January 15, 2006, from http://www.hhs.gov/news/press/2004pres/20040427a.html

HHS. (2005, May 23). *Barriers to adoption.* Retrieved February 20, 2006, from http://www.hhs.gov/healthit/barrierAdpt.html

Institute of Medicine. (1990). *Medicare: A strategy for quality assurance.* Washington, DC: National Academy Press.

Institute of Medicine. (2001). *Crossing the quality chasm: a new health system for the 21st Century.* Washington, DC: National Academy Press.

Iversen, T. (2004). The effects of a patient shortage on general practitioners' future income and list of patients. *Journal of Health Economics, 23*(4), 673–694.

JCAHO. (2006). *A Journey Through the History of the Joint Commission.* Retrieved August 28, 2006, from http://www.jointcommission.org/AboutUs/joint_commission_history.htm

Jencks, S. F. (2004). *The QIO program: legal foundation, recent history and current directions.* Retrieved December 12, 2005, from http://www.medqic.org/dcs/Blob Server?blobcol=urldata&blobheader=application%2Fpdf&blobkey=id&blobtable= MungoBlobs&blobwhere=1106669436962

Jha, A. K., Perlin, J. B., Kizer, K. W., & Dudley, R. A. (2003). Effect of the transformation of the Veterans Affairs health care system on the quality of care. *New England Journal of Medicine, 348*(22), 2218–2227.

Juran, J. M., Gryna, F. M., & R. S. Bingham, J. (Eds.). (1974). *Quality control handbook (3rd ed.).* New York: McGraw-Hill.

Kleinke, J. D. (2005). Dot-gov: market failure and the creation of a national health information technology system. *Health Affairs, 24*(5), 1246–1262.

Kohn, J. T., Corrigan, J. M., & Donaldson, M. S. (Eds.). (2000). *To err is human: building a safer health care system.* Washington, DC: Institute of Medicine.

Kolesar, P. J. (1993). The relevance of research on statistical process control to the total quality movement. *Journal of Engineering and Technology Management, 10*(4), 317–338.

Kuhn, H. (2005, March 16). *Pay for performance initiatives.* Retrieved February 28, 2006, from http://www.hhs.gov/asl/testify/t050315a.html

Lehrman, T. D. (2003). Reconsidering medical malpractice reform: the case for arbitration and transparency in non-emergent contexts. *Journal of Health Law, 36*(3), 475–506.

Levin-Scherz, J., DeVita, N., & Timbie, J. (2006). Impact of pay-for-performance contracts and network registry on diabetes and asthma HEDIS(R)Measures in an integrated delivery network. *Medical Care Research and Review, 63*(1_suppl), 14S–28.

Lien, H. M., Albert, Ma C. T., & McGuire, T. G. (2004). Provider-client interactions and quantity of health care use. *Journal of Health Economics, 23*(6), 1261–1283.

Lillrank, P. (2002). The broom and nonroutine processes: a metaphor for understanding variability in organizations. *Knowledge and Process Management, 9*(3), 143–148].

Lillrank, P. (2003). The quality of standard, routine and nonroutine processes. *Organization Studies, 24*(2), 215.

Lillrank, P., & Holopainen, S. (1998). Reengineering for business option value. *Journal of Organizational Change Management, 11*(3), 246.

Lillrank, P., & Liukko, M. (2004). Standard, routine and non-routine processes in health care. *International Journal of Health Care Quality Assurance Incorporating Leadership in Health Services, 17*(1), 39–46.

Lohr, K. (1990a). IOM study urges a major shift in QA strategy. *QA Review, 2*(5), 1, 7–8.

Lohr, K. (Ed.). (1990b). *Medicare: a strategy for quality assurance*. Washington, DC: National Academy Press.

Luce, J. M., Bindman, A. B., & Lee, P. R. (1994). A brief history of health care quality assessment and improvement in the United States. *West J Med, 160*(3), 263–268.

Marley, K. A., Collier, D. A., & Goldstein, S. M. (2004). The role of clinical and process quality in achieving patient satisfaction in hospitals. *Decision Sciences, 35*(3), 349–369.

McAdam, R., & Corrigan, M. (2001). Re-engineering in public sector health care: A telecommunications case study. *International Journal of Health Care Quality Assurance, 14*(5), 218–227.

McNeil, B. J. (2001). Hidden barriers to improvement in the quality of care. *New England Journal of Medicine, 345*(22), 1612–1620.

McQueen, L., Mittman, B. S., & Demakis, J. G. (2004). Overview of the Veterans Health Administration (VHA) Quality Enhancement Research Initiative (QUERI). *Journal of the American Medical Informatics Association, 11*(5), 339–343.

Middleton, B. (2005). Achieving U.S. health information technology adoption: the need for a third hand. *Health Affairs, 24*(5), 1269–1272.

Nahra, T. A., Reiter, K. L., Hirth, R. A., Shermer, J. E., & Wheeler, J. R. C. (2006). Cost-effectiveness of hospital pay-for-performance incentives. *Medical Care Research and Review, 63*(1_suppl), 49S–72.

Nicholls, S. J., McElduff, P., Dobson, A. J., Jamrozik, K. D., Hobbs, M. S. T., & Leitch, J. W. (2001). Underuse of beta-blockers following myocardial infarction: a tale of two cities. *Internal Medicine Journal, 31*(7), 391–396.

Ortiz, E., Meyer, G., & Burstin, H. (2002). Clinical informatics and patient safety at the Agency for Healthcare Research and Quality. *Journal of the American Medical Informatics Association, 9*(90061), S2–7.

Pawlson, L. G., & O'Kane, M. E. (2004). Malpractice prevention, patient safety, and quality of care: a critical linkage. *American Journal of Managed Care, 10*(4), 281–284.

Pay for performance works, says CMS . . . (2006). *Healthcare Financial Management, 60*(1), 17–18.

Perrow, C. (1984). *Normal accidents: Living with high-risk technologies*. New York: Basic Books.

Plochg, T., & Klazinga, N. S. (2002). Community-based integrated care: myth or must? *International Journal for Quality in Health Care, 14*(2), 91–101.

Poon, E. G., Jha, A. K., Christino, M., Honour, M. M., Fernandopulle, R., Middleton, B., et al. (2006). Assessing the level of healthcare information technology adoption in the United States: a snapshot. *BMC Medical Informatics and Decision Making, 6*, 1. Available from http://www.biomedcentral.com/1472-6947/6/1

Quality directors give QIOs high marks in new study. (2005). *Healthcare Benchmarks and Quality Improvement, 12*(6), 68–69.

Reason, J. (1990). *Human Error.* Cambridge, UK: Cambridge University Press.

Rice, T. H., & Labelle, R. J. (1989). Do physicians induce demand for medical services? *Journal of Health Politics, Policy and Law, 14*(3), 587–600.

Rubenfeld, G. D. (2004). Using computerized medical databases to measure and to improve the quality of intensive care. *Journal of Critical Care, 19*(4), 248–256.

Rubin, R. J., & Mendelson, D. N. (1994). How much does defensive medicine cost? *Journal of American Health Policy, 4*(4), 7–15.

Scalise, D. (2001). Six Sigma: The Quest for Quality. *Hospitals and Health Networks, 75*(12), 41–45.

Schoen, C., Osborn, R., Huynh, P. T., Doty, M., Zapert, K., Peugh, J., et al. (2005). Taking the pulse of health care systems: experiences of patients with health problems in six countries. *Health Affairs,* w5, 509–525.

Schoenbaum, S. C., Audet, A. M., & Davis, K. (2003). Obtaining greater value from health care: the roles of the U.S. government. *Health Affairs, 22*(6), 183–190.

Shewhart, W. A. (1931). *Economic control of quality of manufactured product.* New York: Van Nostrand.

Shewhart, W. A. (1939). *Statistical method from the viewpoint of quality control.* Washington, DC: The Graduate School of the Department of Agriculture.

Shortliffe, E. H. (2005). Strategic action in health information technology: why the obvious has taken so long. Today the United States is poised to achieve what has been sought and anticipated for at least three decades. *Health Affairs, 24*(5), 1222–1233.

Smith, D. C. (1996). The Hippocratic Oath and Modern Medicine. *Journal of the History of Medicine and Allied Sciences, 51*(4), 484–500.

Solberg, L. I., Hurley, J. S., Roberts, M. H., Nelson, W. W., Frost, F. J., Crain, A. L., et al. (2004). Measuring patient safety in ambulatory care: potential for identifying medical group drug-drug interaction rates using claims data. *American Journal of Managed Care, 10*(11 Pt 1), 753–759.

Soumerai, S. B., McLaughlin, T. J., Spiegelman, D., Hertzmark, E., Thibault, G., & Goldman, L. (1997). Adverse outcomes of underuse of beta-blockers in elderly survivors of acute myocardial infarction. *Journal of the American Medical Association, 277*(2), 115–121.

Spiegel, A. D., & Springer, C. R. (1997). Babylonian medicine, managed care and codex hammurabi, circa 1700 b.c. *Journal of Community Health, 22*(1), 69–89.

Sprague, L. (2005). Hospital oversight in Medicare: accreditation and deeming authority. *NHPF Issue Brief, 2005* (802), 1–15.

Steiger, B. (2005). Poll finds physicians very wary of pay-for-performance programs. *Physician Executive, 31*(6), 6–11.

Steinberg, I. (2000). Clinical choices of antibiotics: Judging judicious use. *The American Journal of Managed Care, 6*(23 Supplement), s1178–s1188.

The trouble with re-engineering. (1995). *Management Decision, 33*(3), 39–40.

Viswanathan, H. N., & Salmon, J. W. (2000). Accrediting organizations and quality improvement. *American Journal of Managed Care, 6*(10), 1117–1130.

von Staden, H. (1996). "In a pure and holy way": personal and professional conduct in the Hippocratic Oath? *Journal of the History of Medicine and Allied Sciences, 51*(4), 404–437.

Weber, D. O. (2005). The dark side of P4P. *Physician Executive, 31*(6), 20–25.

Weissman, J. S., Annas, C. L., Epstein, A. M., Schneider, E. C., Clarridge, B., Kirle, et al. (2005). Error reporting and disclosure systems: views from hospital leaders. *Journal of the American Medical Association, 293*(11), 1359–1366.

Wennberg, J. E. (2002). Unwarrented variation in healthcare delivery: Implications for academic medical centres. *British Medical Journal, 325*, 961–964.

Wennberg, J. E. (2005). *Variation in use of Medicare services among regions and selected academic medical centers: is more better?* (No. 874). New York: The Commonwealth Fund.

Wennberg, J. E., & Peters, P. G., Jr. (2004). Unwarranted variations in the quality of health care: can the law help medicine provide a remedy/remedies? *Specialty Law Digest: Health Care Law*(305), 9–25.

Williams, S. C., Schmaltz, S. P., Morton, D. J., Koss, R. G., & Loeb, J. M. (2005). Quality of care in U.S. hospitals as reflected by standardized measures, 2002–2004. *New England Journal of Medicine, 353*(3), 255–264.

Wood, C. (1998). The misplace of litigation in medical practice. *Australian & New Zealand Journal of Obstetrics & Gynaecology, 38*(4), 365–376.

Yasnoff, W. A., Humphreys, B. L., Overhage, J. M., Detmer, D. E., Brennan, P. F., Morris, R. W., et al. (2004). A consensus action agenda for achieving the national health information infrastructure. *Journal of the American Medical Informatics Association, 11*(4), 332–338.

The Strategic Management of Human Resources

Jon M. Thompson

LEARNING OBJECTIVES

By the end of this chapter the student will be able to describe:

- Why human resources management includes strategic and administrative actions;
- Current environmental forces influencing human resources management;
- The key role of employees as drivers of organizational performance;
- Major federal legislation affecting human resources management;
- Human resources functions that address employee workforce planning/recruitment, and employee retention;
- The key responsibilities of human resources management staff and line management staff in recruitment and retention;
- Methods of compensating employees;
- Methods of evaluating employees by using employee performance appraisals; and,
- Examples of human resource management issues in healthcare settings.

INTRODUCTION

The management of human resources is one of the most important yet challenging responsibilities within health services organizations. Health services organizations need to be high performing organizations, and human resources are considered the most important factor in creating such organizations (Pfeffer, 1998). A high performing health services organization provides high quality services and excellent customer service, is efficient, has high productivity, and is financially sound.

Human resources management involves both administrative and strategic elements. From a strategic perspective, health services organizations compete for labor. They desire an adequate labor supply and the proper mix of quality and committed healthcare professionals to provide needed services. The strategic perspective acknowledges that organizational performance is contingent on individual human performance. Health services organizations need to view their human resources as a strategic asset that helps create competitive advantage (Becker, Huselid, & Ulrich, 2001). Additionally, organizations must have the capability to understand their current and future manpower needs and develop and implement a clear-cut strategy to meet those needs to achieve the organizational business strategy. Administratively, there are a number of specific functions and action steps that need to be carried out in support of managing the human resources of the health services organization to ensure high levels of performance.

Fundamentally, human resources management addresses the need to ensure that qualified and motivated personnel are available to staff the business units operated by the health services organization (Hernandez, Fottler, & Joiner, 1998). Human resources management encompasses a variety of functions and tasks related to recruiting, retaining, and developing staff in the health services organization. These staff include administrative staff who carry out non-clinical administrative functions such as patient accounting, quality management, and community relations; clinical staff who provide diagnostic, treatment, and rehabilitation services to patients; and support staff who assist in the delivery of clinical, administrative, and other facility services. The human resources activities that support administrative and clinical staff are carried out by dedicated human resources personnel who work in human resources or personnel departments, and are also carried out by line managers who have primary responsibility for directing staff and teams and who are charged with hiring, supervising, evaluating, developing, and when necessary, terminating staff.

Management of human resources is complex, and human resources actions address a variety of issues/situations. Consider the following examples of human resources management in various health services organizations:

- A large physician practice is in need of hiring someone to head up their information management area. The practice has grown from 7 to 23 physicians in the past 5 years, and the practice administrator has realized that the clinical and financial records needs of the practice have outpaced current administrative expertise. The administrator wants to define the job by analyzing job duties and then recruiting personnel to fill the position.
- A large system-affiliated hospital desires to train patient care technicians to assist in direct clinical care of patients. The hospital has experienced a shortage of RNs in the past 3 years, and has found that a multi-disciplinary team approach using patient care technicians will help the organization meet patient and manpower needs. The Vice President of Patient Care desires to know the best way to train.
- An assisted living facility is developing a new position for a marketing specialist, who will be tasked with marketing the facility in an effort to increase its census. The facility administrator desires to conduct a job analysis to determine the specific responsibilities of the marketing specialist's job.
- An ambulatory care clinic plans to add new diagnostic imaging equipment in order to compete for more patients in their service area. The purchase of this equipment raises several questions for the organization, including: What are the specific human resources needed to staff the new technology and are they available? How will the addition of new technology and services impact the operating budget and the achievement of the business strategy of the clinic?

Each of these scenarios provides a good illustration of the diverse nature of human resources activities from both strategic and administrative perspectives and suggests how these activities contribute to the effective performance of the organization.

This chapter provides an overview of the specific activities that take place strategically and administratively to manage the human resources of the health services organization. First, environmental forces affecting the management of human resources in health services organizations will be reviewed. Second, the importance of employees as drivers of organizational performance will be addressed. Key functions within human resources management will then be identified and discussed. Finally, conclusions regarding management of human resources in health services organizations will be presented.

ENVIRONMENTAL FORCES AFFECTING HR MANAGEMENT

There are several key environmental forces that impact the availability and performance of human resources within health services organizations (HSOs) (see Table 3-1). The environment for HSOs is the external space beyond the organization that includes other organizations and influences that impact the organization.

First, declining reimbursements from government payers and other third parties have reduced the revenues coming to HSOs. In efforts to contain their expenses, Medicare and Medicaid programs and private insurance and managed care organizations have reduced their payments on behalf of covered beneficiaries. Declining reimbursements for health services organizations have left HSOs with fewer resources to recruit, compensate, and develop their workforces. Because other organizations in local and regional markets are also competing for the same labor, this has made recruitment and retention of staff more difficult for many HSOs.

Second, the low supply of healthcare workers—particularly highly specialized clinical personnel—has made recruitment of needed healthcare personnel very challenging (Fottler, Ford, & Heaton, 2002). Many areas of

TABLE 3-1 Environmental Forces and Impacts on Human Resources Management

Force	Impact
Declining reimbursement	Less resources to recruit, compensate, and develop workforce
Declining supply of workers	Shortage of skilled workers; changes in recruiting and staffing specialized services; lower satisfaction of workers
Increasing population need	Increased volumes of patients and workload for HSOs
Increasing competition among HSOs	Competition for healthcare workers and pressure for higher wages
External pressure on HSOs for accountability and performance	HR must ensure high performance in HSO

the country have experienced shortages of nursing, diagnostic, and treatment personnel, a phenomenon that has left many HSOs understaffed, requiring remaining staff to work longer hours per week (Shanahan, 1993). This has also contributed to lower levels of staff satisfaction and higher rates of turnover in certain staff positions, which has in turn increased human resources costs to the HSOs (Izzo & Withers, 2002; Shanahan). In addition, recruiting staff members who are highly specialized and who are in short supply tends to raise human resources costs as HSOs have to pay these staff members higher wages and provide other incentives to appeal to these potential workers (Shanahan).

Third, competition among health services organizations has increased dramatically in the past 15 years due to an increase in supply of traditional HSOs, such as hospitals and nursing homes, as well as the influence of newly emerging HSOs, such as retirement communities, assisted living facilities, and ambulatory care programs. HSOs have engaged in service competition and to a lesser degree, price competition, in trying to outperform their rivals. Competition in services and competition for labor has contributed to increased demands on human resources management.

Fourth, the population's needs for health and medical care have increased in the past 2 decades and will continue to grow during the next 25 years as the population ages and baby boomers approach retirement and qualify for Medicare. Older adults require more health services, and therefore, HSOs will require more healthcare workers to care for the increasing volumes of patients served at their facilities. This is further complicated by the fact that much of the current healthcare workforce is nearing retirement age themselves (Burt, 2005). Thus, in the future, health services organizations will be faced with declining workforces due to retirements, on the one hand, and expanded demands from the population, on the other hand. Projections of the future number of healthcare workers show significant opportunities for employment (see Table 3-2). However, this puts HSOs in a difficult situation: additional workers are needed to care for the increased patient workload, while the supply of workers in many categories continues to be low. This creates additional challenges for recruiting as well as retaining HSO staff.

Finally, increasing regulation and scrutiny of health services organizations by external organizations have increased pressures for high quality and high performing organizations. While licensing and accrediting organizations monitor HSO conformance to standards, they also make these performance indicators available to the public, legislators, and other stakeholders. In addition,

TABLE 3-2 Projected Growth in Healthcare Occupations Employment, 2002–2012

Occupation	Total Employment (000's)		2002–2012 Change in Total Employment		2002 Self-Employed Percent	2002–2012 Average Annual Job Openings (000's)		2002 Median Annual Earnings (Dollars)
	2002	2012	Number (000's)	Percent		Due to growth & total replacement needs	Due to growth & net replacement needs	
Physician Assistants	63	94	31	48.9	0.8	8	4	64,670
Physical Therapists	137	185	48	35.3	5.7	18	6	57,330
Emergency Medical Technicians and Paramedics	179	238	59	33.1	0.8	36	8	24,030
Nursing Aides, Orderlies, and Attendants	1,375	1,718	343	24.9	1.6	336	52	19,960
Physicians and Surgeons	583	697	114	19.5	16.9	41	19	Over 138,400
Medical and Clinical Laboratory Technicians	147	176	29	19.4	1.6	22	7	29,040
Registered Nurses	2,284	2,908	623	27.3	1.2	236	110	48,090
Medical and Health Services Managers	244	315	71	29.3	5.3	36	12	61,370

Source: U.S. Bureau of Labor Statistics, 2005.

reimbursement organizations and government payers like Medicare and Medicaid are increasing requirements on HSOs for accountability and performance by mandating reports on quality, morbidity, and mortality, as well as efficiency and costs. For HSOs, this means that human resources management must help the HSO become a high performing, high quality organization that can demonstrate quality processes and outcomes to these external stakeholders. Human resources can help accomplish this by hiring staff that are high quality, retaining those that are high quality, and reinforcing the culture of a high performing organization.

In addition to the noted external factors, internal factors also impact human resources management. Increasingly, senior management of HSOs view human resources in terms of its contribution to the success of the HSO, and look to human resources indicators in their assessment of overall organizational performance (Becker, et al., 2001; Galford, 1998; Griffith, 2000; Pieper, 2005). As they do with other departments and services, HSO senior management wants to see a return on their investment in human resources functions and a contribution to the bottom line (Becker et al.). Although a support function to the core focus of delivery of patient care services, human resources activities are evaluated in terms of the contribution to recruitment, training, and development for staff, as well as employee satisfaction and retention. Therefore, human resources strategies and programs to address recruitment and retention needs are being developed and assessed, not in terms of whether they look good or because other organizations are doing them, but rather because they contribute to the organization's mission and goals for the creation of a high performing, high quality organization.

UNDERSTANDING EMPLOYEES AS DRIVERS OF ORGANIZATIONAL PERFORMANCE

The core services provided by HSOs—patient care services—are highly dependent on the capabilities and expertise of the organization's employees. It has been said that successful business strategy is directly connected to having committed, high-performance employees (Ginter, Swayne, & Duncan, 2002). HSOs are only as good as their employees. Why is this so for health services organizations?

There are three primary reasons why this is the case. First, HSOs are service organizations, unlike traditional businesses or manufacturing firms that make and distribute a specific product. Being a service organization means providing a service that is needed and/or desired by a consumer who decides to take advantage of what the HSO has to offer. Providing services involves doing things to help others, and HSOs require employees who have a desire to help others, a "service orientation" (Fottler, et al., 2002). Second, HSOs are highly specialized service organizations that provide a range of specific services that include inpatient, outpatient, surgical, rehabilitation, diagnostic, therapeutic, and wellness services. To provide these specialized services, healthcare workers need to carry out many highly specialized tasks, and they need to have the proper knowledge, training, and experience to do those tasks well. Finally, because of the variety of services provided in HSOs and the fact that specialized staff provide only specific "pieces" of the overall service experience, healthcare workers from different departments and units must work together to provide a comprehensive service that meets all the needs of each patient (Liberman & Rotarius, 2000). Therefore, staff must work together as teams to ensure that all required services are provided, and that the total needs of the patient or health care client are met. Therefore, teamwork is necessary in order for the HSO to provide the high quality, coordinated, and comprehensive services that are required for it to be a high performing organization.

In essence, all HSO employees need to work together to ensure the best service possible, centered on the patient's needs. Managers, therefore, must be able to hire good people with the proper knowledge, skills, and attitudes and provide them the resources and support necessary to do their jobs effectively and efficiently.

KEY FUNCTIONS OF HUMAN RESOURCES MANAGEMENT

In this section, the major functions within human resources management will be reviewed. The primary areas of human resources management activity include: job analysis; manpower planning; establishing position descriptions; recruitment, selection and hiring employees; orienting new employees; providing training and development; managing compensation and benefits; assessing performance; providing employee assistance services; and offering employee suggestion programs. Typically, these key functions can be collapsed into two major domains called workforce planning/recruitment and employee retention (see Table 3-3). In the discussion below, the reader should note that activities in these two domains are typically car-

TABLE 3-3 **Human Resources Functions**

Function	Related Tasks
Workforce Planning/Recruitment	Job Analysis
	Manpower Planning
	Recruitment, Selection, Negotiation, and Hiring
	Orientation
Employee Retention	Training and Development
	Compensation and Development
	Assessing Performance
	Labor Relations
	Employee Assistance Programs
	Employee Suggestion Programs

ried out by human resources staff professionals who are under the supervision of a Vice President, Director, or Manager of Human Resources. In some HSOs, this office may be called "personnel," but most health services organizations—particularly large HSOs—now have a department or office of human resources which reflects both a strategic and administrative focus.

The human resources department or office develops and maintains all employee policies and procedures that reflect hiring, evaluating, promoting, disciplining, and terminating employees. In addition, policies and procedures related to assessing employee satisfaction, giving employee awards, compensating employees, and providing benefits are also developed and managed by the human resources staff. Furthermore, all employee records are maintained in the human resources office and in the human resources information system.

It should be noted that many federal and state laws impact human resources management in HSOs. There is a lengthy history of federal legislation that has been enacted to protect the rights of individual employees and to ensure non-discrimination in the hiring, disciplining, promoting, compensating, and terminating of employees on the basis of age, sex, religion, color, national origin, or disability. Many states have also enacted specific laws that protect employees. Other employment issues such as sexual harassment, whistleblowing (identifying wrong-doing), and workplace harassment are also addressed under federal and state law and offer employees protection. The legal environment for HSOs related to human resources management is constantly changing, and employers must carry out their activities with full knowledge of applicable laws and emerging rulings from court cases. Table 3-4 provides a summary of key federal legislation impacting human resources management in HSOs.

TABLE 3-4   Key Federal Legislation Affecting Human Resources Management

1935	**National Labor Relations Act** (as amended in 1974). Provides for bargaining units and collective bargaining in hospitals and health services organizations.
1938	**Fair Labor Standards Act** (as amended many times). Employees who are non-exempt from minimum wage and overtime provisions must be paid minimum wage and time and a half for hours beyond 40 hours per week. Special provisions for health services organizations.
1963	**Equal Pay Act.** Prohibits discrepancies in pay between men and women who perform the same job.
1964	**Civil Rights Act** (as amended many times). Prohibits discrimination in screening, hiring, and promotion of individuals based on gender, color, religion, or national origin (Title VII).
1967	**Age Discrimination in Employment Act.** Prohibits employment discrimination against employees age 40 and older.
1970	**Occupational Safety and Health Act.** Requires employers to maintain a safe workplace and adhere to standards specific to healthcare employers.
1973	**Rehabilitation Act.** Protects the rights of handicapped people (physically or mentally impaired) and protects them from discrimination.
1973	**Employee Retirement Income Security Act (ERISA).** Grants protection to employees for retirement benefits to which they are entitled.
1978	**Pregnancy Discrimination Act.** Requires employers to consider pregnancy a "medical condition" and prohibits exclusion of pregnancy in benefits and leave policies.
1986	**Consolidated Omnibus Budget Reconciliation Act (COBRA).** Gives employees and their families the right to continue health insurance coverage for a limited time due to various circumstances such as termination, layoff, death, reduction in hours worked per week, and divorce.
1986	**Immigration Reform and Control Act.** Establishes penalties for employers who knowingly hire illegal aliens.
1986	**Worker Adjustment and Retraining Notification Act.** Requires employers who will make a mass layoff or plant closing to give 60 days advance notice to affected employees.
1990	**Americans With Disabilities Act (ADA).** Gives people with physical and mental disabilities access to public services and requires employers to provide reasonable accommodation for applicants and employees.
1993	**Family Medical and Leave Act (FMLA).** Permits employees in organizations to take up to 12 weeks of unpaid leave each year for family or medical reasons.
2003	**Health Insurance Portability and Accountability Act (HIPAA).** Affords employee protection from outside access to personal health information and limits employers' ability to use employee health information under health insurance plans.

Sources: Lehr, McLean & Smith, 1998; and Busse, 2005.

WORKFORCE PLANNING/RECRUITMENT

Human resources functions carried out within the workforce planning/recruitment domain are directed to analyzing jobs needed within the HSO; identifying current and future staffing needs; establishing position descriptions; recruiting, selecting, negotiating, and hiring employees; and orienting new employees.

Job Analysis

One of the fundamental tasks of human resources is to conduct an analysis of all jobs or positions that are a part of the HSO. Every position in the HSO—whether administrative, support, or clinical—needs to be justified in terms of its specific responsibilities and day-to-day activities. **Job analysis** involves identifying those unique responsibilities, duties, and activities specific to every position in the HSO. This is necessary to clarify individual responsibilities, but is also critical to avoid duplication of tasks and responsibilities across positions. The outcome of job analysis is to clearly state the responsibilities, duties, and tasks of every position within the HSO.

Recent human resources experts have suggested that HSOs should focus on those positions that contribute most directly to the completion of the organization's business objectives (Huselid, Beatty, & Becker, 2005). This is important because filling these critical positions with the best personnel—"A" players—will then increase the organization's ability to perform.

Manpower Planning

For every position established for the HSO, there needs to be an estimate of the number of staff members needed to carry out those responsibilities at the present time, as well as projections of the number of staff members needed at some future target date. For example, how many RNs does our hospital currently need for all the various services that we currently offer, and how many will we need in 5 years? This is a very complex decision process, and must be based on consideration of many factors. For example, consider a hospital. Will the hospital be downsizing or eliminating any services in the next 5 years? Will the facility be adding any new services that are not presently offered? How will the addition of new technology, or the addition of nursing assistants, affect the need for RNs in the future, across all services of the hospital?

Identifying current numbers of staff is based on volume statistics that reflect the current performance of the HSO. The need for clinical staff is based typically on patient care statistics, such as the number of patients admitted, number of outpatient visits, or the number of patients receiving a specific service. In some cases, need will be determined by licensure standards that govern the minimum number of staff for certain services. For non-patient care areas, including such support functions as medical records, information technology, and financial services, the number of staff needed is contingent on the current volume of records and patient accounts that must be processed. Each support person in these areas can handle a minimum number of accounts or records per day, which becomes the basis for estimating current need. This is a called a **ratio method of determining needs**. The managers in various units calculate these estimates and forward them to human resources for the development of aggregate estimates of staffing needs for the total facility.

Projections of staffing needs for a future target date are based on a similar method. Projections of future service volumes are made and associated staffing requirements are projected as well to serve that anticipated volume. Again, line managers usually develop these projections. Future volumes are typically determined through a consensus-based strategic planning process where there is agreement on **future service volumes**. In this process, consideration is also made for retiring staff, transfers, and service changes (such as eliminations or expansions of beds and services) to arrive at the needed number of staff to recruit or to acquire on a temporary basis from outside staffing firms. Once the projected staffing needs are identified for the total facility, strategies and timeframes are established for recruiting. Projections of staffing needs are revisited every year as annual performance is assessed to see if projections remain accurate.

Accuracy of projections has important implications for preparing budgets and evaluating financial performance of the HSO. For example, future staffing levels may be unrealistic if forecast revenues don't match projected expenses. Therefore, planned positions may remain unfilled and flexible staffing arrangements used as necessary. In addition, if demand shifts occur, some services may not realize projected patient volumes and cutbacks in staffing arrangements may be necessary. In conclusion, projections of future staffing requirements are just that—projections that may or may not hold up given the uncertain and dynamic nature of the health services environment. Many factors affect these projections and a thorough and periodic assessment is needed to ensure projections are realistic and revised as appropriate.

Establishing Job Descriptions

Position descriptions or job descriptions are required for every position within the HSO. Job descriptions are necessary to define the required knowledge, skills, responsibilities, training, experience, certification or licensure, and line of reporting for a specific job within the HSO. Such descriptions are important to both the organization and employee. The position description elaborates on the findings from the job analysis and provides a means by which the organization clarifies each position in terms of expectations, locus within the organizational structure, and how it contributes to the organization's overall performance. For the employee, the position description clarifies expectations and duties and allows prospective employees a means to evaluate the "fit" between a position and their own individual knowledge, skills, and experience.

Position descriptions are developed through joint efforts of line managers and human resources staff. Line managers specify job requirements; human resources staff keep job descriptions in a consistent format and ensure accuracy of the positions as they are included in the HSO's Human Resources Information System. An example of a position description for a hospital is shown in Figure 3-1.

Recruitment, Selection, Negotiation and Hiring of New Employees

A key principle of human resources recruitment is making sure that HSO positions are filled with competent and highly skilled personnel. Once recruitment needs are made known by line managers, it is the responsibility of human resources to follow the appropriate procedures to fill those positions. In some cases, existing employees will have an interest in a new position for which they are qualified, and internal candidates will be considered. Human resources recruitment personnel use a standard process for external recruiting. These steps include advertising, screening applicants, determining those to be interviewed, conducting interviews, selecting the candidate, negotiating, and hiring. Activities for both human resources staff and line managers related to recruitment are identified in Table 3-5.

BON SECOURS HEALTH CORPORATION
St. Francis Medical Center

POSITION DESCRIPTION

TITLE:	**Environmental Services Aide**	**JOB CODE: 950**
DEPARTMENT:	**Environmental Services**	
REPORTS TO:		**FLSA: Non-exempt**

I. GENERAL PURPOSE OF POSITION:

The primary responsibility of this position is to perform cleaning tasks to maintain designated areas in a clean, safe, orderly and attractive manner. The employee is expected to follow detailed instructions and/or written task schedules to accomplish assigned duties. This position serves all populations of visitors, employees, physicians and patients.

II. EMPLOYMENT QUALIFICATIONS:

1. Ability to communicate and interpret assignments issued through a computerized paging system.
2. Dependability and flexibility demonstrated through previous work or school history.
3. Previous housekeeping work experience preferred.

III. ESSENTIAL JOB FUNCTIONS:

1. Communicates all hospital-related issues to Supervisor.
2. Performs the duties necessary to maintain the sanitary conditions of the hospital, including routine cleaning and maintenance of all floor types.
3. Prepares patient rooms for new admissions through the proper utilization of the Bedtracking® system. (Login\Logout)
4. Cleans and sanitizes isolation rooms and other contaminated areas following written techniques appropriate for that type of isolation (i.e., tuberculosis, HIV, hepatitis).
5. Performs general cleaning tasks using the 7 Steps process.
6. Follows hospital policy regarding storage and security of housekeeping chemicals.
7. Accurately uses Bedtracking® system to meet departmental response and cleaning time standards.
8. Responsible for the use and care of equipment and other hospital property. Maintains equipment by proper cleaning and storage; reports dangerous or broken equipment to team leader. Makes sure EVS cart is clean, box locks, and wringer free of lint.
9. Understands basic safety procedures. (RACE, PASS, MSDS, etc.)

IV. OTHER JOB EXPECTATIONS:

1. Actively participates in the hospital's Continuing Educational Improvement programs (i.e., Essential Skills, Safety Fairs, etc.)
2. Assists in the orientation of new employees in departmental methods and procedures.
3. Responds to unusual occurrences such as flood, spillage, etc.

V. WORKING CONDITIONS:

Works in all areas of the hospital and off-site properties. May be exposed to hazardous chemicals, but potential for harm is limited, if safety precautions are followed.

The individual performing this job may reasonably come into contact with human blood and other potentially infectious materials. The individual in this position is required to exercise universal precautions, use personal protective equipment and devices, when necessary, and learn the policies concerning infection control.

VI. BON SECOURS MISSION, VALUES, CUSTOMER ORIENTATION AND CONTINUOUS QUALITY IMPROVEMENT FOCUS:

It is the responsibility of all employees to learn and utilize continous quality improvement principles in their daily work.

All employees are responsible for extending the mission and values of the Sisters of Bon Secours by understanding each customer, treating each patient, staff member, and community member in a dignified manner with respect, kindness, and understanding, and subscribing to the organization's commitment to quality and service.

VII. APPROVALS   DATE

Department Manager

Administration _____

Human Resources

The above statements are intended to describe the nature and level of work being done by individuals assigned to this classification and are not to be construed as an exhaustive list of all job duties. This document does not create an employment contract, and employment with Bon Secours Richmond Health System is "at will".

_____

Source: Reprinted with permission from Bon Secours St. Francis Medical Center, Midlothian, Virginia.

FIGURE 3-1 Position Description

TABLE 3-5 **Responsibilities of HR Staff and Line Managers in Recruitment**

HR Staff Person

Prepares Position Description

Does job pricing

Prepares advertisements/recruitment materials

Keeps track of applicants/maintains HR Information System

Checks applicant references

Maintains personnel files

Narrows candidate pool

Line Manager

Clarifies job function/provides input into Position Description

Interviews candidates

Ranks candidates

Selects candidate

Negotiates with candidate

Hires candidate

Advertising

Different modes of advertising are used to target candidates and generate interest. These sources include local newspapers and electronic media including radio and television, organizational web sites, and Internet job search engines, e.g., www.monster.com and CareerBuilder.com. The human resources department uses standards for communication that address the position, required degrees, training and/or certification, experience, functional line of reporting and general expectations of the position. Applicants submit information in response to the advertising and submit their credentials that are reviewed and evaluated by human resources staff.

Candidates are recruited also through private recruitment or "headhunter" firms, and these may include firms that engage in general staff recruiting or firms that specialize in health services organization staff by recruiting nurses, technicians, financial analysts, or office personnel. Arrangements with recruiters usually involve paying a percentage of the first year salary to the recruiter if the candidate referred by the recruitment firm is selected for the position. This method of recruiting will result in costs that exceed the normal expected costs of filling position vacancies. However, this technique may be a necessary option when recruiting for highly specialized positions where the candidate pool is limited.

Another frequently used option in recruiting is to work with educational programs that prepare specialized health personnel, such as nurses, physical therapists, and diagnostic technicians (Shanahan, 1993). Sending announcements of positions to these educational programs, attending recruitment open houses, and developing important referral relationships with faculty and staff of these programs are helpful in building interest and identifying candidates. Other sources include placing ads in targeted professional journals that are read by healthcare professionals, disseminating recruitment materials to healthcare workers identified through association membership listings, and attending regional or annual meetings of professionals where human resources representatives can meet with interested candidates. A final option to identify interested candidates is for human resources staff to attend healthcare recruitment or job fairs held locally or regionally, or for the HSO to hold its own.

Some observers have suggested that HSOs use a pre-employment assessment by the candidate of the fit between their credentials and the job (Liberman & Rotarius, 2000). This is recommended to ensure that only appropriate, well-qualified applicants apply.

Interviewing, Selection, Negotiation, and Hiring

Human resources staff complete the preliminary review and analysis of candidates based on their applications, check candidate references, and identify past employers' satisfaction with the candidates. As a result, human resources staff narrow the pool down to those candidates that provide the best fit for the position based on training, experience, and other factors such as motivation and attitude. These applicants are then discussed with the line manager to select those to be interviewed. The candidates are invited to come to the organization and interview and spend some time with management, staff, and others. From the HSO's perspective, this is important for two reasons. It enables the HSO to assess first-hand the candidates and verify their knowledge and skills; also, it enables the assessment of the candidates' fit and compatibility with the organization and staff with whom they would be working. From the candidate's perspective, an interview is important to get a close look at the organization and staff, and to assess their fit and interest in the position and the organization.

Depending on the position, human resources staff may participate in candidate interviews, and line managers will definitely participate in interviews with candidates. Structured interviews with clearly defined questions are thought to be best for assessing candidates (Foster & Godkin, 1998). Subsequent to the interviews, the staff who have interviewed candidates meet to review the candidates, determine how the candidates match with position requirements and rank order candidates. Once the staff agree on the applicant they would like to hire, an offer is extended.

An offer of employment is made in writing and the offer letter must specify the position for which the offer is made, start date, associated salary/compensation and benefits, and any other key information regarding the offer. Although an offer has been extended, the recruitment process is not complete. Depending on the position, there may be a period of negotiation over salary, benefits, start time, flexible scheduling, and other issues. Once agreement is reached, the position is assumed filled and the candidate responds with a formal letter of acceptance agreeing to the position and conditions of acceptance. Completion of hiring paperwork is necessary at the time that the person starts the job. It should be noted that if agreement is not reached with the first choice candidate, then the offer would be extended to the next best candidate, and then the next, until agreement with a suitable candidate is reached.

Orientation

One of the key requirements of a new staff member is to attend an orientation program coordinated by human resources. This program is important for several reasons. An orientation program informs the new employee of policies, procedures, and requirements, and it offers an opportunity for the new employee to ask questions and clarify understanding about the organization. The **Employee Staff Manual** is provided to each new employee. During orientation, various policies and procedures are highlighted, including expectations for the work day, proper attire and behavior, employee assessment, disciplinary actions and grievances, probationary period, and opportunities for training and development. The organization's values, mission, vision, and goals are reviewed, as are strategic and long-range plans. Specific employee benefits are identified and reviewed, and employees are informed about options concerning benefits and associated costs. Safety and security policies and practices are reviewed, and in large HSOs such as hospitals and nursing homes, special codes are revealed so that employees know when and how to respond to emergency situations such as fires, patient medical emergencies, patient problems, intruders, and chemical and environmental emergencies. With the passage of the Health Insurance Portability and Accountability Act (HIPAA) in 1996, training in the requirements of this law regarding confidentiality of health information has been incorporated into many HSO's employee orientation sessions. Training in compliance with Medicare rules and regulations, along with the dissemination of Whistleblower Protection Act information is also becoming a part of new employee orientation in many HSOs.

Orientation is usually held once a month to coincide with the start date for new employees. Part-time, full-time, and short-term temporary employees are typically required to attend orientation. New employees have an opportunity to meet the senior management team, who typically provide an overview of their respective management domains during orientation. This helps new staff gain an understanding of their respective roles in the HSO.

EMPLOYEE RETENTION

Employee retention functions include all of those key activities that address care, support, and development of employees to facilitate their long-term commitment to the organization. The key functions under employee retention include training and development, managing compensation and benefits, assessing performance, providing employee assistance programs, and offering employee suggestion programs.

Training and Development

Training and development of the workforce are extremely important human resources functions for several reasons. First, the organization's need for specific knowledge and skills is always changing because of the rapid changes being experienced by HSOs. For example, HSOs frequently add new medical technologies that require different technical skills of employees. Another example of additional skills needed is in the information technology area, where new computer information systems, electronic medical records, databases, and integrated patient and financial data systems are being acquired to generate, store, and retrieve patient-level and organizational information. Second, training is necessary to provide for continuing education of some staff. For clinical staff that require continuing education as part of their licensure and/or certification, HSOs may coordinate the provision of training that is provided either on site or at remote locations. While it is clear that not all the training and develop-ment needs of staff can be met due to resource limitations, the human re-sources staff determines priorities for annual training and education efforts and implements and manages those programs. Human resources staff typ-ically accomplish this through organization-wide needs assessments or through identification of specific training needs that are made known to human resources staff by managers. Typically, the cost of training and de-velopment programs is provided for in the human resources budget; in some cases, other departments or services within the HSOs may cover the cost of training that is coordinated by human resources.

The goal of any training or development effort is to provide value for the organization by returning benefits, such as increased productivity, greater effectiveness, higher quality, greater coordination of care, and en-hanced patient or customer service. Therefore, training and development programs are evaluated by human resources for cost-effectiveness to ensure that training was effective in terms of return on investment, and that methods of training were appropriate (Phillips, 1996). Training programs cover a range of topics, including technical training on equipment and software programs, customer service training, and training to improve inter-personal communications and leadership, among others. Training and development of teams within HSOs are also increasingly common, as HSO staff work frequently in teams to coordinate the delivery of care. The effectiveness of team leaders has been shown to influence team learning, development, and performance (Edmonson, Bohmer, & Pisano, 2004).

Managing Compensation and Benefits

The following sections describe the management of employee compensa-tion and benefits in healthcare organizations and how it can contribute to a high-performing organization.

Compensation

The human resources department has the specific responsibility of man-aging the pay or compensation and benefits associated with all positions held within the HSO. This is no easy task, as specific pay ranges and ben-efits must be established for each position, which in the hospital industry includes over 300 distinct jobs or major job classifications (Metzger, 2004). The management of compensation begins with a clear definition of the HSO's compensation philosophy, which reflects the organization's mission, values, and strategy regarding human resources, as well as consideration of internal (e.g., equity) and external (e.g., competitive) factors (Gering & Conner, 2002; Joiner, Jones, & Dye, 1998).

Determining compensation refers to the establishing of a specific financial value for a job. Compensation for each position is set based on the consideration of a number of factors, including the specialized knowledge and skills associated with the position, the experience required for the position, the relative availability of skilled individuals to fill the position, and average wages that are specific to the local labor market. This is called "job pricing" (Joiner et al., 1998). Some positions are **hourly rated** (i.e., non-exempt, and eligible for overtime pay), where a compensation rate per hour of work is established (e.g., for maintenance staff and floor nurses), and some positions are salaried (i.e, exempt and not paid overtime), where an annual salary is paid the employee (e.g., nurse managers and other managerial staff). In short, compensation is set to account for the special skills and experiences required of employees and to enable the organization to be competitive in the market in securing and retaining needed employees. Pay ranges will vary by type of position, but within a position class there must be equity. However, HSOs typically account for differences in training, experience and special considerations of the job (working weekends or evenings) by allowing for pay/shift differentials. Also, some jobs are subject to significant external market pricing, because the skill set is unique and the market is national or international.

The typical large HSO, such as a hospital or hospital system, has a separate, designated staff to handle the administration of compensation, on the one hand, and benefits, on the other. Human resources staff responsible for compensation keep records of wages and salaries, compensation adjustments, and the basis for compensation adjustments in individual employee personnel files and in the Human Resources Information System. Every few years, human resources administers a compensation or salary survey for positions within the HSO in order to **benchmark** current compensation to local and regional market trend (i.e., a comparative market analysis of wages), and adjust salary ranges for positions as appropriate to remain competitive.

Job pricing is used to establish equitable pay scales by position within HSOs, but reward systems beyond base pay are frequently considered of greater importance to employees (Joiner et al., 1998). In addition to base compensation tied to expectations for a specific job, many HSOs have embraced incentive compensation. While compensation plans focus on individual performance and allocating rewards such as raises to high performers based on individual performance, incentive plans are designed to improve organizational performance (Gibson, 1995). In an **incentive** or **pay-for-performance plan**, the purpose of the plan is to stimulate employees to higher levels of achievement and performance that benefits the organization. Meaningful measures such as profits (return on investments), productivity, attendance, safety, quality, and customer satisfaction are a few examples of financial, as well as non-financial organization-wide, performance indicators that can be used in developing incentive plans. The incentive plan would work in the following way. The organization would set target goals for performance in a specific time period. At the end of that time period, the organization would collect and review relevant information to measure the status of performance. If the measurement of performance on specific indicators met the target goals, the organization would then reward employees for the "organization-wide" performance. These programs are also known as **gainsharing** or **goal-sharing programs**, and payouts (revenues derived from savings, increased productivity or volumes, increased customer retention, and quality) would be shared with employees as a bonus for their contributions to high performance within the HSO (Gomez-Mejia, Welbourne, & Wiseman, 2000).

Incentive compensation plans have long been thought to be associated with higher levels of organizational performance (Bonner & Sprinkle, 2002). The theory behind this approach is that use of incentives such as compensation bonuses positively affects motivation which leads to higher performance (Gibson, 2002). Many health services organizations have begun to follow the lead of business and industry who pioneered these programs, but published literature addressing the impact of incentive compensation on organizational performance in healthcare is limited (Griffith & White, 2002). There is some recent evidence to show that more HSOs are using incentive programs for executives that are tied to organizational performance (HMFA, 2001). However, recent research in the business literature has shown that the relationship between incentive pay and performance may not hold up.

Beer and Katz (2003) found in their survey of senior executives from among many firms that bonuses have little to no positive effect on performance, and that their real function may be to attract and retain executives. They looked at firms that had implemented executive bonus compensation systems and assessed relationships to performance, but found that the only key explanatory factor was that the incentive system promoted *teamwork*. Similarly, Luthans and Stajkovic (1999) found in their analysis of research on pay-for-performance that social recognition and administrative feedback to employees on performance were just as influential as pay-for-performance in achieving higher levels of performance in a manufacturing setting. Moreover, Beer and Cannon (2004) found that many senior managers view incentive compensation programs with concern, and question whether the benefits outweigh the costs. However, none of the studies cited above were specific to health services organizations.

Benefits

The human resources staff is responsible for managing benefits provided to employees working in an HSO. A benefit is defined as any type of compensation provided in a form other than salary or direct wages, that is paid for totally or in part by an employer (Jenks & Zevnik, 1993). As benefits extended to workers in general have increased over the past two decades, the number and type of benefits made available to HSO employees have increased as well (Griffith & White, 2002; Runy, 2003). However, the HSO is faced with a dilemma. On the one hand, HSOs are under pressure to manage costs, and employee benefits have been a high cost item for HSOs, which directly affects the HSO's cost management strategy, financial status, and competitive position. On the other hand, benefits as a portion of total compensation have increased in importance, as more and more employees indicate that benefits are important in their choice of an employer (Runy).

Benefits may differ by level within the organization, as management may receive one set of benefits to offset the higher level of skill needed to complete the job, versus lower level employees who may receive fewer benefits due to a lower level of skills required for the job. The availability of benefits, as well as the percentage of employee cost sharing, varies widely by HSO. However, typical benefits offered by HSOs include the following:

Sick leave. A certain number of days per year are allocated for the employee being unable to be on the job due to illness or injury.
Vacation. A certain number of vacation days are allocated to employees for them to use as free time. In many HSOs, this is combined under a **Paid-time-off (PTO)** plan with sick leave days and holidays.

Holidays. Designated national holidays are given to employees with pay as part of their benefits.

Health insurance. Medical coverage for the employee and optional coverage for dependents are typically made available. Depending on the type of health insurance plan offered to employees (and there may be one or more plans offered by the HSO), the total plan cost for the employee may be shared by the employer and employee. HSOs, like other organizations, have turned to managed care plans as a way to reduce health benefits expense for the HSO. Typical plan features include greater cost-sharing and out-of-pocket expenses for employees, along with the trend of increased access to out-of-network and specialty care. In addition, much of the coverage by health insurers today focuses on the management of certain chronic clinical conditions, such as cardiovascular problems and diabetes. These **disease management programs** are offered in an attempt to help the employee and dependent manage their conditions to promote better quality of life and reduce cost.

Life Insurance. Coverage is provided that will help offset the loss of earnings for a limited time and to cover burial and other expenses related to the death of an employee. The employee is typically provided a base amount of life insurance with an option to increase coverage for an additional cost.

Flexible health benefits. Flexible or "cafeteria" benefits are increasing in popularity as they are offered to employees as options. Flexible benefits most often include health insurance, dental insurance, eye coverage, and other health benefits such as disability insurance and long-term care insurance, where the employee is granted a choice in benefits for specific costs. Flexible benefits offer advantages to the employee in that the employee can tailor benefits to meet individual needs at varying costs (Joiner et al., 1998). For the HSO, overall benefit costs can be reduced under flexible benefit plans due to the fact that the employer is no longer paying for a specific base package of benefits for all employees (Joiner et al.).

Retirement benefits. Many HSOs have retirement plans in place where employees are granted a certain percentage of their compensation over and above their compensation that is put into a retirement fund. This fund can be a pension fund that is set up specific to the HSO or more likely, a 401(k) or 403(b) plan where employees can manage their retirement dollars in mutual fund investments (Jenks & Zevnik, 1993). Many HSOs also have included the option in the retirement plan of offering to "match" employees' contribution to the plan with employer-paid funds up to a maximum amount. Retirement funds can only be accessed at the age of retirement or fund withdrawals are subject to penalties.

Flexible Spending Accounts. These are also called reimbursement accounts, and are offered by the HSO to help the employee and their dependents by allowing pre-tax dollars to be placed into a healthcare or dependent care account. These accounts are then used to pay for costs incurred by the employee and dependents that are not covered under other benefits plans or for the care of a child or dependent, disabled parent (Jenks & Zevnik, 1993).

Other benefits. Several other categories of benefits are also made available to HSO employees, although the degree to which they are offered and the scope of coverage will vary considerably. These benefits may include personal health benefits (complementary and alternative healthcare, yoga and pilates classes, wellness/fitness center memberships, health education programs, and personal health risk appraisals); transportation (use of a van pool); educational reimbursement (tuition for employee or dependent's college); employee incentives (profit sharing, stock options); flexible work scheduling, job-sharing and telecommuting; child care assistance and on-site child care; and savings programs (matched savings plans), among many others (Jenks & Zevnik, 1993).

Occupational safety and health. The Human Resource Department contributes to the organization's efforts to maintain a safe and healthy work environment. Responsibilities are carried out in several ways to address this concern. First, **workers' compensation coverage** is required for organizations under state law, in order to protect workers who may get sick due to the job or become injured or incapacitated due to working conditions. This coverage is separate from any health insurance provided. Second, the HSO monitors federal and state regulations for occupational safety and monitors risk in the organization and works to eliminate safety risks. Sometimes these human resources staff activities are conducted in conjunction with the risk management activities within the HSO.

Employee Assistance Programs

Employee Assistance Programs (EAPs) are HSO-sponsored programs that are made available to employees, and in many cases their dependents, to assist with personal or family problems that also affect the employee's job performance (Howard & Szczerbacki, 1998). Such problems include stress and mental health problems, family dysfunction and divorce, alcohol and substance abuse problems, financial problems, legal issues, and adjustment issues stemming from a death in the family, loss of a job, or severe illness. In addition, the patient care services provided in an HSO are often challenging and stressful, and providing care to individuals who are sick, injured, and in some cases dying or near death, is very trying and stress inducing for employees (Blair, 1985). This may lead to feelings of helplessness, guilt, or grief that negatively impact attendance and threaten the employee's focus, effectiveness, and productivity. Workplace stress may also be exacerbated by personal and family stress outside the HSO. As a result, HSOs have recognized the value of EAPs to help employees in their times of need, by making available counseling, stress reduction programs, health education programs, and other interventions based on need to lessen the impact of these problems. A problem-free, happy employee is an employee who is more likely to be focused and productive on the job. This results in positive performance for the individual employee as well as the HSO. The cost of services to the employee will vary depending on how the EAP is structured; some of the needed EAP services may be covered under other current employee benefits. EAP services can be offered on-site at the HSO or offered at remote locations under contract with other providers, which facilitates greater confidentiality for users. Employees are also afforded protection from harassment and job loss due to use of the EAP.

In summary, the benefit package has become more important to employees in recent years as employees balance tradeoffs between compensation and an appropriate array of benefits that are important to the employee and dependents. For example, many employees with young families may be more interested in a broad range of benefits, such as those discussed above, rather than the highest salary possible. Such benefits help employees meet their own unique needs, and become a significant factor in employee recruitment and retention. In the end, benefits may be one of

Management Summary Form

Confidential

Development Level:
1 = Performs below standard
2 = Inconsistently meets the standard
3 = Consistently meets the standard
4 = Frequently exceeds the standard
5 = Consistently exceeds the standard

.... Annual Review
.... Other

(For the initial review, please use the "Introductory Performance Review" Form)

Instructions: The Performance Improvement Plan is a tool designed to assist in managing, developing and reviewing an employee's effectiveness and efficiency. It also provides a common understanding of job expectations for present and future performance review periods. *Please note all supporting comments on the Development Plan.*

I. Values (includes integration of Quest for Excellence Behaviors) *(see page 6-7 of the Process Guide)*

		Developmental Level				
A.	Respect - commitment to treat people well (e.g., responsive - returns calls/emails).	1	2	3	4	5
	Justice - supporting and protecting the rights of all people.					
	Integrity - honest in dealings (e.g., honors commitments, keeps promises).					
	Compassion - experiencing empathy with another's life situation.					
B.	Stewardship - responsible use of Bon Secours resources (e.g., consistently on time).	1	2	3	4	5
	Innovation - creating or managing new ideas, methods, processes and/or technologies.					
	Quality - continuous improvement of service; involved in Gallup/Quest planning.					
	Growth - developing and improving services and promoting self-renewal; completion of previous year's Development Plan. (e.g., thinks "Big Picture").					

Average Developmental Level for Section I (A + B/2):

II. Leadership Competencies (see page 10-14 of the Process Guide)

	Developmental Level				
Change Management & Organization Development - planning & designing change strategies as needed; integrating individual dev. & organizational dev. into strategies.	1	2	3	4	5
Communication & Interpersonal Skills - listening & responding in constructive manner; promoting understanding while building productive working relationships.	1	2	3	4	5
Critical Thinking - examining underlying causes & determining best course of action.	1	2	3	4	5
Human Resource Development - facilitating others to achieve professional dev. goals.	1	2	3	4	5
Planning & Strategic Direction Setting - determining shape of present & future job environment; efficiently maintaining & improving practices; setting direction for dept./org.; **developing Gallup Impact, PRC, Quest for Excellence Plans.**	1	2	3	4	5
Promotion of Mission & Values - setting an example by integrating org. standards into day-to-day functions; guiding others to a common Mission & Vision.	1	2	3	4	5
Self-Knowledge & Insight - using personal understanding to promote positive self-change.	1	2	3	4	5
Team Building - promoting teamwork to accomplish dept./org. objectives.	1	2	3	4	5
Proficiency in Field - subject matter expert in field; resource to others.	1	2	3	4	5

Average Developmental Level for Section II (Sum of 9 Leadership Competency Dev. Levels/9):

III. Essential Job Functions
    (This section is determined by the Job Description and will vary with the Position being evaluated)

Average Developmental Level for Section III:

Overall Average: *(Average Level for Section I x .5) + (Average Level for Section II x .25) + (Average Level for Section III x .25)*

FIGURE 3-2 Performance Evaluation

Development Plan

Name: _____

Facility & Dept.: _____

The Purpose of the Development Plan is to aid in the process of developing specific skills and behaviors. The Plan is reviewed and finalized during the performance review meeting. At a minimum, progress towards reaching agreed upon goals should be discussed once during the year. *This form must be completed by each employee and returned prior to the performance review.*

1 **Previous Objectives, Goals and Accomplishments.** Review learning and development objectives, goals and accomplishments achieved since last performance review; include knowledge and skill strengths used to accomplish objectives and goals.

2 **New Objectives and Goals.** Identify new learning and development objectives and goals for he coming year, which include addressing opportunities for growth. Include issues, which may need to be addressed and opportunities needed to successfully implement, including implementation of Quest/Team Player improvements.

3 **Employee and/or Manager's Comments.** Additional comments may be made on a separate sheet of paper and attached to this form.

FIGURE 3-2 (continued) Performance Evaluation

the most critical factors in making the HSO competitive in attracting and retaining staff.

Assessing Employee Performance

The human resources department is charged with developing and maintaining a system for measuring employee performance for all employees of the HSO. The central theme of this chapter is that organizational performance is paramount and that individual employee performance in an HSO is highly contributory to organization-wide performance. Therefore, assessing individual employee performance is critical to understanding and achieving high levels of organizational performance.

Under human resources department leadership, a **Performance Appraisal System** is established for the HSO. **Performance appraisal** means assessing the performance of an individual employee. In order for the HSO to know how individuals are performing and to develop a plan and program for employees to improve performance, an annual performance assessment is required. The assessment form includes several criteria that are determined to be important for the HSO in evaluating performance. These criteria may include measures of both quality and quantity of the work as specified in the position description and include technical skill assessment, as well as other criteria that address the employee's motivation, attitude, and interpersonal skills in carrying out their respective work. Human resources, in conjunction with senior management of the HSO, will determine what specific criteria are included in the performance appraisal. Performance appraisals also include an assessment of the degree to which an individual's annual goals and objectives have been achieved as spelled out in the yearly management plan. See Figure 3-2 for an example of a Performance Appraisal used by Bon Secours-St. Francis Hospital.

Kirkpatrick (2006) argues that a performance appraisal system must be part of the organization's efforts for continuously improving performance. Performance assessment is conducted by line managers for their subordinates on an annual basis, at the time of the employee's anniversary date or more commonly, at a standard time to coincide with the budget development process for the upcoming year. Using the agreed upon form, the manager will complete an assessment of each subordinate's performance for the assessment period. The manager then will sit down with the employee and review the appraisal and discuss areas of favorable performance, as well as areas of improvement opportunity. This will also give the subordinate an opportunity to express any concerns and/or seek clarification as to the basis for the evaluation ratings. Many managers also ask subordinates to complete a self-evaluation for the performance period under review, using the same criteria, for discussion at the meeting. It should be noted that good managers communicate with their subordinates about employee performance regularly throughout the year, with an interest in monitoring, correcting, and improving performance on an on-going basis.

At the designated annual performance appraisal meeting between a manager and a subordinate, a meaningful exchange can be carried out in order to frankly discuss performance, identify opportunities for improving performance, and developing a specific plan for achieving higher levels of performance. A two-way discussion of these matters is the most fruitful for both parties, as the employee will understand the manager's concern and interest in the employee and the sincere desire for improving performance. In addition, the employee can express likes and dislikes about the job, which the manager needs to know (Butler & Waldroop, 2005). However, it is essential that clarity be provided in communicating performance as perceived by the supervisor, so that there is no confusion as to the intent of the evaluation (Timmreck, 1998). A key outcome of the performance evaluation is the setting of **performance improvement goals**, actions to achieve the improvements, and priorities for action (Kirkpatrick, 2006). In addition to an annual performance appraisal, the HSO may require some or all employees to be reviewed for satisfactory performance at the end of their first 90 days of employment (often referred to as the **probationary period**), and at other times as specifically requested by a manager or if conditions warrant.

Performance appraisals are helpful to management and employees in the following ways (Longest, Rakich, & Darr, 2000):

- The manager can compare absolute as well as relative performance of staff;
- Together, the manager and employee can determine a plan for improving performance if such improvement is needed;
- Together, the manager and employee can determine what additional training and development activities are needed to boost employee performance;
- The manager can use the findings to clarify employee desires to move up to higher level positions and/or expand responsibilities;

- The manager can document performance in those cases where termination or reassignment is necessary;
- The manager can determine adjustments to compensation based on performance; and,
- The manager can determine promotional or other advancement opportunities for the employee.

In addition to the traditional method of assessing performance described above, many HSOs are now employing **360-degree performance appraisal systems.** While this method also includes a manager-subordinate evaluation, it provides for multisource feedback on employee performance from a number of other stakeholders—including peers, the employee's subordinates and internal and external customers, if applicable. Feedback is aggregated and communicated to the employee through a neutral third party such as a human resources staff member. The advantages to using the 360-degree evaluation are reduction of fear of repercussion from evaluative comments and a greater range of feedback from a larger number of observers of the employee/manager (Garman, Tyler, & Darnall, 2004). However, there are some disadvantages as well. These include the higher cost of administration of a 360-degree evaluation compared to a traditional evaluation, and the lack of an instrument suitable for health services managers (Garman et al.). In addition, peer feedback included in 360-degreee evaluation may also be biased or inaccurately given, due to difficulties in determining an individual's contribution to the unit or service, or fear of providing negative feedback to a colleague (Peiperl, 2005).

One of the most challenging outcomes of the performance appraisal process is the need to terminate an employee. Although the goal of human resources management is to retain high performing staff, not all employees will be retained. There are many reasons why an employee can be discharged, but in every case the primary reason must relate to performance deficiency. Terminating an employee is not easy and is uncomfortable at times for managers who have the authority to discharge an employee. However, failure to act decisively will jeopardize the HSO's performance and will certainly reflect negatively on the manager's ability as a leader (Hoffman, 2005). In situations where an employee is not likely to be retained, it is essential that the manager not wait until the appraisal to assess the employee's performance. In fact, ongoing monitoring of performance, efforts to correct performance problems, and documentation of the steps taken in any corrective processes are all typically required prior to discharge. This process should be done by the line manager in close consultation with the human resources manager. The HSO policies and procedures must be adhered to carefully to prevent subsequent allegations of wrongful discharge, and potentially avert a lawsuit against the HSO and/or the line manager.

Managing Labor Relations

Labor relations is a general term that addresses the relationships between staff (labor) and management within HSOs. Labor relations is associated with **collective bargaining** where a union, if certified (i.e, voted in by the workers), represents the interests of employees who become members of that union. Nationally, about 20% of HSOs have at least one union represented in their organizations (Longest et al., 2000). In the period 1980–1994, there were 4,224 certification elections held in health services organizations: 31% of these were in hospitals, 40% in nursing homes, and 29% were in other healthcare facilities (Scott & Lowery, 1994). Union elections in health services organizations vary by type of healthcare setting, but overall about 60% of elections result in a union being approved (Deshpande, 2002). Unions have a higher than average win rate in hospitals, and hospitals have been the focus of increased union organizing efforts in recent years (Deshpande, 2003).

Why do unions get involved in HSOs? As seen in manufacturing, the fundamental reason for unionization in health care is that employees are dissatisfied with some aspects of the work and/or the work environment, and feel that management is insensitive to their needs. Unions often step in where management has failed to do its job. If staff are strongly dissatisfied with various aspects of the HSO, view senior management as poor communicators, and/or perceive that management is insensitive to staff issues, they may believe that a union is the only way to have their voice heard and needs met. If elected to represent employees in an HSO, a union is then authorized to engage in collective bargaining with management of the HSO regarding wages, working conditions, promotion policies, and many other aspects of work (Longest et al., 2000).

The National Labor Relations Act of 1935, as amended, enables union organizing and collective bargaining in health services organizations. The Act also created **The National Labor Relations Board (NLRB)**, which recognizes several bargaining units for healthcare employees, including nurses, physicians, other professional employees, and non-professional employees, among others. The NLRB has the authority to oversee and certify the results of union elections. There are many rules and regulations that must be followed in unionization activity, and there are certain restrictions placed on management as well as staff that govern what can and cannot happen regarding union discussions, organizing and elections.

The presence of a union creates significant challenges for management of an HSO. From management's perspective, unions create an unnecessary third party in decisions that affect the employment relationship and work of the HSO's staff, which raises potential for conflict. Union requirements may restrict the administrator's ability to use the number and type of staff in desired ways, and compensation negotiated by the union may reduce management's ability to directly control staffing expenses. Labor unions can also limit an HSO's discretionary authority to make changes in the workplace and in workplace practices (Holley, Jennings, & Wolters, 2001). Also, some research has shown that productivity may be negatively affected after unionization (Holley et al.).

Beyond general impact on administration, unionization has been shown to significantly affect the human resources function in HSOs. Deshpande (2002) found in a study of hospital unionization activity that the presence of unions resulted in higher numbers of employees who were screened, a higher number of employee training programs, a greater number of job classifications, greater use of employee performance appraisal methods, and lower productivity, as reported by CEOs of hospitals.

Various strategies have been discussed with respect to the administrative stance vis-a-vis unions (Deshpande, 2003). To reduce the possibility of union discussions and union organizing, administrators are encouraged to keep communication open and fluid, provide competitive salaries and benefits, establish grievance policies and procedures, and ensure staff participation and involvement in decision-making as much as possible. In all respects, administrators and human resources staff should continuously assess staff satisfaction and needs, as well as opportunities for staff and management to work together for the better of the organization and larger community. There are many challenging issues that affect HSOs, including lowered reimbursements from managed care and government payers, cost reduction practices, and lower staffing ratios. These can lead to employee dissatisfaction, and management needs to be cognizant of the negative impact of some of their decisions on staff motivation, satisfaction, and commitment.

If one or more unions are certified to represent employees in an HSO, then much of the time and effort of the human resources staff will be spent in addressing unionization issues. These include negotiating (bargaining) aspects of the union contract, ensuring that specific aspects of the contract are met, communicating with union representatives, and being the focal party in carrying out all union discussion and negotiation under the auspices of federal labor law (Longest et al., 2000).

Employee Suggestion Programs

Employee suggestion programs (ESPs) are increasingly being considered by HSOs in an effort to encourage creativity on the part of employees and to identify needed improvements in processes and outcomes. Employee suggestion programs have been in existence for quite some time (Carrier, 1998), but the primary locus has been in manufacturing and other business enterprises as opposed to HSOs.

An ESP works simplistically by soliciting employee suggestions for change and acknowledging and rewarding those suggestions that offer the most potential to meet organizational goals and implementing those suggestions. These programs usually are formally structured, widely communicated throughout the organization, and managed by human resources staff. Current ESPs have gone far beyond the old suggestion box model and include elements of electronic submission and web-based applications, as well as formal recognition and reward (Fairbank, Spangler, & Williams, 2003).

ESPs are part of an overall effort by HSOs to stimulate innovation and creativity for ideas that will help the HSO. The underlying rationale for the program is that employees of HSOs, as key providers of its services and activities, are in the best position to know what can be improved and may have good ideas as to how such improvements can be made. ESPs are built on the premise that innovation in organizations can be understood from a problem-solving approach (Fairbank et al., 2003). Goals of ESPs can include organizational improvements, such as reducing costs, improving methods and procedures, improving productivity, improving equipment, and cutting waste, as well as increasing job satisfaction and organizational commitment on the part of employees (Carrier, 1998). This second goal of ESPs is very important and should not be overlooked by the human resources staff. Part of the overall satisfaction in working in an HSO is the belief that management understands and appreciates its employees, and is interested in their input. ESPs are not, however, without their limitations. Drawbacks to the program include difficulties in designing a program, effectively administering it, and sustaining the program over several years. (Kim, 2005).

CONCLUSION

The management of human resources is an important function within HSOs because the performance of HSOs is tied directly to the motivation, commitment, knowledge, and skills of clinical, administrative, and support staff. Human resources actions of HSOs are undertaken for both strategic and administrative purposes. A variety of human resources activities are included within the human resources area, and these activities typically fall within the domains of workforce planning/recruitment and employee retention. While human resources serves as a support function for line managers within HSOs, line managers and staff managers carry out human resources management roles as well, because they are involved in hiring, supervising, evaluating, promoting, and terminating staff. Therefore, human resources staff and other managers work closely to ensure that HSOs perform well. The contribution of the human resources management function is increasingly being evaluated by senior management, similar to other organizational functions, to determine the net contribution of human resources staff to organizational success. It is likely that management of human resources will increase in importance in the future, as HSOs face heightened external and internal pressures to recruit and retain committed and high performing staff.

DISCUSSION QUESTIONS

1. Describe why human resources management is comprised of strategic and administrative actions.

2. For each human resources scenario described in the introduction to the chapter, identify the steps you would take to address the specific human resources issue being faced. From your perspective, which is the most challenging issue, and why?

3. Two key domains of human resources management are workforce planning/recruitment and employee retention. Describe several human resources functions that fall under each and describe their importance to human resources management.

4. Identify and describe some environmental forces that affect human resources functions in health services organizations.

5. Define and contrast "Employee Assistance Programs" and "Employee Suggestion Programs."

6. Why do HSOs offer incentive compensation programs? How do these programs differ from base compensation programs?

REFERENCES

Becker, B. E., Huselid, M. A., & Ulrich, D. (2001). *The HR scorecard.* Boston: Harvard Business School Press, 2001.

Beer, M., & Cannon, M. D. (2004, Spring). Promise and peril in implementing pay-for-performance. *Human Resources Management, 43*(1), 3–48.

Beer, M., & Katz, N. (2003). Do incentives work? The perceptions of a worldwide sample of senior executives. *Human Resource Planning, 26*(3), 30–44.

Blair, B. (1985). *Hospital Employee Assistance Programs.* Chicago: American Hospital Publishing, Inc.

Bonner, S. E., & Sprinkle, G. B. (2002). The effects of monetary incentives on effort and task performance: Theories, evidence and a framework for research. *Accounting, Organizations and Society, 27*, 303–345.

Burt, T. (2005, November/December). Leadership development as corporate strategy: Using talent reviews to improve senior management. *Healthcare Executive, 20*(6), 14–18.

Busse, R. C. (2005). *Your rights at work.* Naperville, IL: Sphinx Publishing.

Butler, T., & Waldroop, J. (2005). Job sculpting: The art of retaining your best people. In *Appraising employee performance* (pp. 111–136). Boston: Harvard Business School Press.

Carrier, C. (1998, June). Employee creativity and suggestion programs: An empirical study. *Creativity and Innovation Management, 7*(2), 162–72.

Deshpande, S. P. (2002). The impact of union elections on human resources management practices in hospitals. *Health Care Manager, 20*(4), 27–35.

Deshpande, S. P. (2003). Labor relations strategies and tactics in hospital elections. *Health Care Manager, 22*(1), 52–55.

Edmondson, A., Bohmer, R., & Pisano, G. (2004). Speeding Up Team Learning. In Harvard Business Review on *Teams that Succeed* (pp. 77–97). Boston: Harvard Business School Publishing Corporation.

Fairbank, J. F., Spangler, W. E., & Williams, S. D. (2003, Sept/Oct). Motivating creativity through a computer-mediated employee suggestion management system. *Behavior and Information Technology, 22*(5), 305–314.

Foster, C., & Godkin, L. (1998, Winter). Employment selection in health care: The case for structured interviewing. *Health Care Management Review, 23*(1), 46–51.

Fottler, M. D., Ford, R. C., & Heaton, C. (2002). *Achieving Service Excellence: Strategies for Healthcare*. Chicago: Health Administration Press.

Galford, R. (1998, March/April). Why doesn't this HR department get any respect? *Harvard Business Review, 76*(2), 24–32.

Garman, A. N., Tyler, J. L., & Darnall, J. S. (2004, Sept/Oct). Development and validation of a 360-degree-feedback instrument for healthcare administrators. *Journal of Healthcare Management, 49*(5), 307–322.

Gering, J., & Conner, J. (2002, November). A strategic approach to employee retention. *Healthcare Financial Management, 56*(11), 40–44.

Gibson, V. M. (1995, February). The new employee reward system. *Management Review, 84*(2), 13–18.

Ginter, P. M., Swayne, L. E., & Duncan, W. J. (2002). *Strategic management of health care organizations* (4th ed). Malden, MA: Blackwell Publishers, Inc.

Gomez-Mejia, L. R., Welbourne, T. M., & Wiseman, R. M. (2000). The role of risk sharing and risk taking under gainsharing. *Academy of Management Review, 25*(3), 492–507.

Griffith, J. R. (2000, Jan/Feb). Championship management for healthcare organizations. *Journal of Healthcare Management, 45*(1), 17–31.

Griffith, J. R., & White, K. R. (2002). *The well-managed healthcare organization* (5th ed). Chicago: Health Administration Press/AUPHA Press.

Healthcare Financial Management Association (HFMA). (2001, August). More healthcare organizations using quality measures to reward executives. *Healthcare Financial Management Association, 55*(8), 22–25.

Hernandez, S. R., Fottler, M. D., & Joiner, C. L. (1998). Integrating management and human resources. In Fottler, M. D., Hernandez, S. R., & Joiner, C. L. (Eds). *Essentials of Human Resources Management in Health Services Organizations*. Albany, NY: Delmar Publishers.

Hoffman, P. B. (2005, Nov/Dec). Confronting management incompetence. *Healthcare Executive, 20*(6), 28–30.

Holley, W. H. Jr., Jennings, K.M., & Wolters, R. S. (2001). *The labor relations process* (7th ed.). Orlando, FL: Harcourt College Publishers.

Howard, J. C., & Szczerbacki, D. (1998). Employee assistance programs in the hospital industry. *Health Care Management Review, 13*(2), 73–79.

Huselid, M. A., Beatty, R. W., & Becker, B. E. (2005, Dec). 'A Players' or 'A Positions'? The logic of workforce management. *Harvard Business Review*, 110–117.

Izzo, J. B., & Withers, P. (2002). Winning employee-retention strategies for today's healthcare organizations. *Healthcare Financial Management, 56*(6), 52–57.

Jenks, J. M., & Zevnik, B. L. P. (1993). *Employee benefits*. New York: Collier Books/Macmillan Publishing Company.

Joiner, C. L., Jones, K. N., & Dye, C. F. (1998). Compensation management. In Fottler, M. D., Hernandez, S. R., & Joiner, C. L. (Eds) *Essentials of human resources management in health services organizations*. Albany, NY: Delmar Publishers.

Kim, Dong-One. (2005, July). The benefits and costs of employee suggestions under gainsharing. *Industrial and Labor Relations Review, 58*(4), 631–652.

Kirkpatrick, D. L. (2006). *Improving employee performance through appraisal and coaching* (2nd ed.). New York: American Management Association/AMACOM.

Lehr, R. I., McLean, R. A., & Smith, G. L. (1998). The legal and economic environment. In Fottler, M. D., Hernandez, S. R., & Joiner, C. L. (Eds). *Essentials of human resources management in health services organizations*. Albany, NY: Delmar Publishers.

Liberman, A., & Rotarius, T. (2000, June). Pre-employment decision-trees: Jobs applicant self-election. *The Health Care Manager, 18*(4), 48–54.

Longest, B. B., Rakich, J. S., & Darr, K. (2000). *Managing health services organizations and systems*. Baltimore: Health Professions Press.

Luthans, F., & Stajkovic, A. D. (1999, May). Reinforce for performance: The need to go beyond pay and even rewards. *The Academy of Management Executive, 13*(2), 49–57.

Metzger, N. (2004). Human resources management in organized delivery systems. In Wolper, L. F. (Ed). *Health care administration* (4th ed.). Sudbury, MA: Jones and Bartlett Publishers.

Peiperl, M. A. (2005). Getting 360-degree feedback right. In *Appraising employee performance* (pp. 69–109). Boston: Harvard Business School Press.

Pieper, S. K. (2005, May/June). Reading the right signals: How to strategically manage with scorecards. *Healthcare Executive, 20*(3), 9–14.

Pfeffer, J. (1998). *The human equation*. Boston: Harvard Business School Press.

Phillips, J. (1996, Apr). How much is the training worth? *Training and Development, 50*(4), 20–24.

Runy, L. A. (2003, Aug). Retirement benefits as a recruitment tool. *Hospitals and Health Networks, 77*(8), 43–49.

Scott, C., & Lowery, C. M. (1994, Winter).Union election activity in the health care industry. *Health Care Management Review, 19*(1), 18–27.

Shanahan, M. (1993). A comparative analysis of recruitment and retention of health care professionals. *Health Care Management Review, 18*(3), 41–51.

Timmreck, T. C. (1998, Summer). Developing successful performance appraisals through choosing appropriate words to effectively describe work. *Health Care Management Review, 23*(3), 48–57.

U.S. Department of Labor, Bureau of Labor Statistics. (2005). 2002 Employment and Wage Estimates and Projections Between 2002 and 2012. Retrieved April 27, 2005 from www.bls.gov

Umiker's Management Skills for the New Health Care Supervisor

Fifth Edition

Charles R. McConnell, MBA, CM
Human Resources and Health Care
Management Consultant
Ontario, New York

JONES AND BARTLETT PUBLISHERS
Sudbury, Massachusetts
BOSTON   TORONTO   LONDON   SINGAPORE

Chapter 4

Customer Service

It is not the employer who pays the wages.
Employers only handle the money. It is the
customer who pays the wages.

—Henry Ford

CHAPTER OBJECTIVES

- Develop an understanding of what the various customers served by the healthcare organization and its employees need from their relationship with healthcare provider organizations.
- Briefly describe the impact of managed care on the delivery of services to the customers of the organization.
- Identify the essential elements of customer service.
- Address techniques that can be applied in improving the personnel systems so important in providing and sustaining superior customer service.
- Identify the elements of an effective customer satisfaction system.

WHO ARE OUR CUSTOMERS AND WHAT DO THEY WANT?

Any activity in any business has both external and internal customers. Customers external to healthcare organizations include patients, patients' families and visitors, referring physicians, doctors' offices, blood donors, and third-party payers. Internal customers include nurses, staff physicians and other professionals, students, trainees, employees, departments, and committees.

There is a distinct difference between a person's wants and that individual's genuine needs. As the widow in the retirement home said, "I need a husband; I want

121

Tom Selleck." Patients are ordinarily aware of their wants. By and large they want quiet, clean rooms with all the conveniences of a first-rate hotel. They want tasty food served hot and on time. They want painless procedures and no waiting on gurneys or in ready rooms. They want courteous, attentive, skillful, and professional-looking staff. Most of all, they want to leave the institution alive and feeling better than when they arrived. On the other hand, few patients are completely aware of their needs for diagnostic tests or therapeutic modalities.

Physicians are not always cognizant of what they should order for their patients until they learn about some new diagnostic or therapeutic procedure. Then they demand it. They invariably want fast and courteous service and all the latest technology.

Insightful care providers take steps to determine what their customers must have (their needs), what they want, and what they do not want. To stimulate or modify the needs and wants of their customers, healthcare providers make their customers aware of new services or products as they become available. What they often forget to do is find out what new services or products their external customers want or need.

INFLUENCE OF MANAGED CARE

The shift to managed care has had considerable impact on customer service. In terms of their effects on customers, managed care organizations—such as health maintenance organizations and preferred provider organizations—have placed certain restrictions on access to care. Government and insurers have forced providers to find ways of operating on less money than they might have received in the absence of managed care. Provider organizations have had to adjust to the financial limitations imposed on them. As a result the healthcare industry has experienced numerous mergers and affiliations and other forms of restructuring, making it necessary to tighten staffing overall at precisely the same time managed care is forcing an increase in customer service communication with an increasing number of internal and external customers.

Under managed care, for the first time in the history of American health care, significant restrictions have been placed on the use of healthcare services. Customers have been introduced to the use of the primary care physician as the "gatekeeper" to control access to specialists and other services. Under the gatekeeper concept, visits to specialists and certain others are covered only if the patient is referred by his or her primary care physician. Before the advent of managed care one could safely say that the acute care hospital was the center of the healthcare system. Now, however, in the role of gatekeeper it is the primary care physician who functions as the practical center of the healthcare system.

As managed care continues to mature and individuals gain more experience in dealing with it, enrollees are becoming more sophisticated in their knowledge of what is promised and what is delivered. Many persons are increasingly critical of how they are handled, especially concerning real and perceived barriers to their access to medical specialists and expensive procedures. Customer inquiries and complaints are on average becoming more complex and articulate and thus more difficult to address.

Although all agencies claim that quality care and patient satisfaction remain important, the emphasis on cost control and limitation of services is unmistakable. Managed care has been directly or indirectly responsible for staff reductions and for the replacement of numerous highly trained personnel with employees who have been educated to a lesser level and thus are paid less.

The impact of managed care is not likely to diminish in the foreseeable future. Many people depend on managed care plans. During late 1998 and 1999, some 160 million Americans were enrolled in managed care plans, and although overall managed care participation seems not to have grown appreciably since then, neither has it diminished. Present membership may represent the overwhelming majority of people suitable for managed care. In-and-out participation of some groups, such as the younger aging and Medicaid patients, is expected, but the bulk of people on whom managed care plans can best make their money are already enrolled.

THREE ESSENTIALS OF CUSTOMER SERVICE

The essentials of customer service in any activity in which employees deal directly with customers are systems, strategies, and employees.

Systems

Systems include policies, protocols, procedures, arrangement and accessibility of the physical facilities, staffing, operations, workflow, and performance monitoring. Policy statements and procedure manuals provide behavior guidelines, rules, and regulations. For effective and customer-friendly policies, several things must be done:

1. Eliminate policies that adversely affect client satisfaction (for example, unnecessarily strict visiting hours).
2. Annually review all policies affecting customer service.
3. Establish a committee of supervisors and knowledgeable employees to address policy matters.
4. Introduce new policies that improve client service (for example, a special parking area for blood donors, more convenient locations and times for specimen collections).

For each new service that is introduced, consider a policy specific to that service.

Discussions in subsequent chapters address policies relating to personnel selection, orientation and training, reward systems, communication, empowering people, and building teams.

Strategies

Strategy in customer service consists of developing a customer-oriented culture. A customer-oriented culture is achieved when every employee understands that good service is expected, that exceptional service is rewarded, and that unsatisfactory service is not tolerated. Such strategy involves statements of vision, values, mission, goals, objectives, and action plans.

Customer feedback is essential to strategy. We obtain feedback from a number of sources, including complaints, suggestions, incident reports, surveys, interdepartmental meetings, cross-functional work groups, task forces, and focus groups.

Employees

We can never forget our internal customers. Employees in all capacities are our best customers in that we must satisfy them before we can please other customers. A well-satisfied employee is one who is capable of extending the best in customer service to others. Concerning employee satisfaction, the principal personnel responsibilities of supervisors are to

1. Determine and respond to the legitimate needs and wants of their employees.
2. Field the best possible team of employees.
3. Empower employees to solve problems (can each of your employees say "I rarely need anyone else to help me handle customer problems or questions"?).
4. Teach by example.
5. Insist on excellent customer service and constantly monitor the delivery of this service.

TECHNIQUES FOR IMPROVING PERSONNEL SYSTEMS

Position Descriptions

In the summary statement of every position description the word "customer" should appear, with an indication of how the customer is to be regarded. (For example, "The goal of this position is to meet or exceed customer expectations and needs. Our external and internal customers include . . . .")

Modify performance standards to include items addressing quality and customer service. Here are some examples:

- Exercises discretion with patient information
- Accepts night and weekend assignments willingly
- Displays tact in personal interactions with customers and staff
- Frequently reports customer comments and suggestions

Recruiting Process

Your goal should be to hire employees who are competent, caring, and resistant to turnover. Assist in the recruiting process by providing the employment section of your human resources department with concise, up-to-date position descriptions. Be sure the attractive aspects of each job are prominent in those descriptions. Help the recruiters by recommending the most effective means for identifying potential job candidates. Answer inquiries about jobs enthusiastically, and interview candidates promptly.

Selection Process

Hire for attitude, train for skill.

The ability to sell jobs to candidates is important. The stronger the candidates appear to be, the more likely it is that other organizations will be trying to hire them. You can learn a great deal about a candidate's attitude toward customer service by asking the following questions: What does superior service mean to you? What gives you the strongest feeling of satisfaction about your workday? Provide an example of how you made an extra effort to serve a client.

Orientation and Training System

Make certain that new employees know who their external and internal customers are. Orient them toward exceptional customer service. Infuse them with the latest ideas in quality improvement. Emphasize the importance of a "can do" attitude and how this can affect performance ratings. Review workflow and carefully address each point at which the providers and recipients of service come into direct contact. Alert new employees to questions that customers frequently ask, and let them know where the answers can be found. Describe what you regard as proper telephone and electronic communication etiquette. Introduce them to the department's major customers.

Performance Review and Reward Systems

Refocus performance objectives and performance appraisals to strongly address customer satisfaction. Discuss customer service when reviewing past performance and when formulating objectives for future activities. Encourage employees to set objectives such as attending seminars on communication skills or customer service, visiting internal customers, or learning to speak customers' languages.

Tie your recognition and reward strategy to customer service. Unfortunately, the healthcare personnel who have the most client contact are among the lowest paid, receive the least training, and have the least opportunity for promotion.

Inservice Educational Programs

Inservice education topics for all employees should include customer identification, recognition of customer expectations, customer problem solving, presenting new services, and communication skills, telephone courtesy in particular. Topics for employees responsible for contact with customers should also include empathic interactions, listening skills, dealing with complaints, assertiveness, and how to cope with angry people.

Personnel Retention

Turnover of personnel presents a major impediment to customer service. Unfortunately, the employees who provide most hands-on service experience the highest turnover rates.

DESIGNING A CUSTOMER SATISFACTION SYSTEM

Principles of effective customer service for supervisor and employees include the following:

- Always treat customers as you would like to be treated.
- Anticipate your customers' needs and wants.
- Hire employees who have a caring attitude, and retrain, reassign, or get rid of those who do not.
- Include customer satisfaction in your orientation and training programs.
- Make yourself a model of good customer service.
- Make customer satisfaction a condition of satisfactory performance.
- Monitor the behavior of your service providers, and coach those who demonstrate any deficiencies.
- Obtain frequent feedback from internal and external customers.
- Underpromise and overdeliver; whenever possible give customers more than they expect.
- Work the right way the first time.

- Recognize and reward those who make special efforts to please customers.
- Give your employees the authority to resolve customer complaints.

Address Complaints

Patients are most likely to complain about noise, food, their rooms, waiting, and lack of courtesy. Customers are displeased when

- They do not receive what is expected or promised.
- They have to wait for what they consider excessive amounts of time.
- Someone who represents the organization is rude, patronizing, or indifferent.
- They believe they are getting the brush-off or the runaround.
- Someone expresses a "We can't do it" attitude or hits them with the rule book (for example, "It's our policy").

Always regard complaints as suggestions for improving service. Some complaints are not legitimate, but a great many are. Legitimate or otherwise, an employee's initial response to any complaint should be careful listening. Complaints are the least costly source of customer feedback. Invite additional comments and ask for specific suggestions for improvement. Encourage your staff to report complaints and make suggestions for eliminating them, and record these suggestions. Express your appreciation of these suggestions at performance reviews as well as at the time they are offered.

Ask for customer comments and suggestions at every staff meeting. Suggestions need not be elaborate or complicated. In one large hospital, for example, music was piped into the waiting room for visitors, most of whom were waiting for patients undergoing surgery. The results of a study of this practice indicated that self-reported stress levels of visitors were reduced.[1]

Maintain a comment log. Empower your front-line troops to solve customer problems. Most customers are understanding if they believe that providers care about them, so give your employees the authority they need.

When faced with a complaint, acknowledge its validity and offer an apology as appropriate. Accept responsibility without blaming others. Empathize with the complainers and ask them what they would like done. If you receive no response, make an offer. Thank the person for bringing the matter to your attention. Promise to do what you agreed to do, then do it promptly.

Think About It

A satisfied customer is your best advertisement. The customer who believes he or she received good service may or may not tell others about the experience, but you can be certain that the customer who received poor service will tell others, perhaps many.

Questions for Review and Discussion

1. Why is it necessary to concern ourselves with internal customers?
2. Why are employees our best customers?
3. How would you respond to customer demands that were clearly unreasonable?
4. Why do you suppose hospital patients are likely to complain most about food, cleanliness, and staff treatment rather than about the quality of care?
5. Do you believe managed care has made customer service more difficult? Why or why not?
6. How are the quality of health care and excellence in customer service related to each other?
7. How does present-day customer service relate to the increasing tendency toward competition among healthcare providers?
8. Is employee turnover ever a significant barrier to good customer service? Why or why not?
9. What do you believe has the greatest influence on an employee's willingness to deliver excellent customer service?
10. Relative to customer service, why is it suggested that we "underpromise" and "overdeliver"?

Exercise: Identifying Customers and Their Needs

Designate a specific healthcare organization function or department (for example, nursing service, physical therapy, housekeeping, or food service). Make it the one you presently work in or one you have worked in at one time. If you are not experienced, select any function or department with which you are comfortable.

Create two blocks of space on a sheet of paper, upper half and lower half, and label one "Internal Customers" and the other "External Customers" (with "internal" and "external" referring to the organization, not just the department—in other words, employees of another department remain your "internal" customers). In each half-page space list as many internal and external customers as you can for your designated department. Next, for each customer designation write a one-sentence description of the services you provide to that customer. If this exercise is done in a classroom setting, compare your lists with others and attempt to reconcile any differences that arise.

Case: The Crabby Receptionist

"I don't know what I'm going to do about Louise," said section supervisor Missy Clare to her friend and fellow supervisor, Janet Stevens. "She was a good worker for the longest time, but now I'm getting complaints."

Janet asked, "What kinds of complaints?"

"That she's brusque to the point of rudeness when she answers the phone and that she snaps at other employees when they just ask simple questions. I've had at least three doctors tell me I'd better get someone more pleasant out front, and obviously someone complained to Carson—you know, my boss—because he asked me about the crabby receptionist in my section he was hearing about."

"Has she been experiencing any kind of problem that you know of? Something personal that's bothering her?"

"I don't know," Missy answered, "and it's a cinch she doesn't want to talk about it even if there is a problem. I've given her every opportunity to talk but she's not having any of it."

Janet said, "Well, to be completely honest with you, I've heard a few things about Louise."

"Like what?"

"Like how some of your outpatients are afraid to approach her because they don't know if they're going to be snapped at, glared at, or ignored."

Missy said, "Louise is such a long-time employee I hate to just lower the boom on her."

"Well, kiddo," said Janet, "you'd better lower something before Carson and his higher-ups get any more complaints."

Questions

1. How would you go about trying to balance the customer service needs of the section with the apparent needs of Louise, the long-time employee?
2. Which of the section's customers are likely to cause Missy the most grief over Louise's behavior? Why?
3. Recommend an approach for Missy to consider in addressing the problem with Louise.

REFERENCES

1. Routhieaux, R. L., and D. A. Tansik. 1997. The benefits of music in hospital waiting rooms. *Health Care Supervisor* 16:31–39.

RECOMMENDED READING

K. Albrecht and R. Zemke, *Service America* (Homewood, IL: Dow Jones-Irwin, 1985).
J. Carlzon, *Moments of Truth* (Cambridge, MA: Ballinger, 1987).

R. Y. Chang and P. K. Kelly, *Satisfying Internal Customers First* (Irving, CA: Richard Chang Publishers, 1994).

W. H. Davidow and B. Uttal, *Total Customer Service* (New York, NY: Harper & Row, 1989).

R. L. Desatnick, *Managing to Keep the Customer* (San Francisco, CA: Jossey-Bass Publishers, 1988).

L. Goldzimer, *"I'm First." Your Customer's Message to You* (New York, NY: Rawson, 1989).

W. Umiker, *The Customer-Oriented Laboratory,* 2nd ed. (Chicago, IL: ASCP Press, 1997).

Chapter 5

Planning

Great success in any enterprise comes from a
balanced combination of three elements:
the mission, the leadership, and the people
who make it happen. By far the most
important is the mission.

—Roger Dawson[1]

CHAPTER OBJECTIVES

- Establish the benefits of planning and convey an understanding of the implications of the failure to plan.
- Provide familiarization with the types of plans used in business activity and identify and explain the key elements of planning.
- Establish the role of planning in an organization's vision and mission.
- Establish the significance of goals and objectives in planning.
- Define action plans and examine the elements of a typical action plan.

Planning is the most fundamental of the management functions, and as such it logically precedes all other functions. Planning is the projection of actions intended to reach specific goals. In other words, a plan is a blueprint for the future; it is our expression of what we wish to accomplish or our best prediction of what might occur in the future. Planning begins with the questions of what and why, then focuses on the how, when, who, and where.

BENEFITS OF PLANNING

Planning ensures that we work effectively and efficiently or at least improves our chances of doing so. Planning reduces procrastination, ensures continuity, and provides for more intelligent use of resources. Planning improves our chances of doing things right the first time, reducing the chances of false starts and resulting in the satisfaction of having everything under control at present and knowing what to do next.

Planning is proactive. It decreases the need to manage from crisis to crisis. It is a prerequisite for practically all necessary managerial activities, including teaching or mentoring, preparing for and running committee and staff meetings, conducting performance appraisal discussions or employment interviews, preparing budgets, and numerous other activities. Planning is essential for coping with crises such as fires, natural disasters, strikes, bomb threats, or hostage incidents.

Because plans work out exactly as anticipated only once in a while, why bother? Isn't planning just effort that's wasted, consuming time that could be better spent acting and doing? Perhaps those whose thinking runs along such lines feel uneasy because they can see the amount of time spent in planning but are uneasily aware that nothing concrete is happening during that time to advance the completion of the work. However, those who discount the value of planning often discover that without planning their efforts are wasted on false starts and misdirection such that excess time is consumed in setting things right.

If things often do not happen exactly as we planned for them to happen, what have we gained by planning? We have been able to apply our efforts more effectively than without a plan, and even though we might not have hit the target precisely, we nevertheless have acquired some important information. As a result we know by how much the target was missed, and we can proceed to determine whether (1) we need to readjust our direction to attain the target or (2) conditions have changed such that the target should be adjusted. In any case, the effort expended in planning is never wasted.

We have all undoubtedly heard the expression, "If we fail to plan, we plan to fail." This is largely true. Without planning, even that which does get done suffers to an extent because it has consumed more time and effort than necessary, and without direction established through planning, the pursuit of any particular result can be an expensive journey into chaos.

CLASSIFICATIONS OF PLANS

Strategic plans are plans made for achieving long-range goals and living up to the expectations expressed in statements of mission and values. Without strategic planning, few visions are realized. *Tactical plans* translate broad strategies into specific objectives and action plans.

Organizational plans begin with a table of organization. They include position descriptions, staffing, and channels of communication. *Physical plans* concern topography (for example, the site of a building, the layout of an office, or the location of diagnostic and therapeutic equipment).

Functional plans are plans concerned with the workings of major functional units such as a nursing service, clinical laboratory, human resources department, financial or clinical services, and others. *Operational plans* address systems, work processes, procedures, quality control, safety, and other supportive activities. *Financial plans* address the inflow and outflow of money, profit and loss, budgets, cost and profit centers, charges, and salaries.

Career planning, *time management*, and *daily work planning* are also vital forms of planning. Daily work planning, the simplest, most elementary form of planning in the working world, frequently proves to be the form of planning most immediately beneficial to the individual supervisor.

KEY ELEMENTS OF PLANNING

The essential elements of planning are vision, mission, goals, objectives, strategy, and action.

Vision

> *A vision is an image without great detail. It acts as a*
> *flag around which the troops will rally.*
>
> —M. Hammer and J. Champy[2]

Vision statements and mission statements deal with purpose and alignment at an organizational level. Without these, the energy of an organization can become scattered rather than focused. Leaders create a vision around which people rally, and managers marshal the resources to pursue that vision. Vision provides a premise that leaders commit to and dramatize to others. A vision statement should not read like a financial report or a concise statement of purpose. Rather, an effective vision statement must tap peoples' emotions; it must conjure up a compelling positive vision that fires people up. Martin Luther King, Jr., provided the best and simplest example of a vision statement with his "I have a dream" speech.

An organization's vision statement should be clear and exciting and should leave broad latitude for the pursuit of new opportunities. The vision of top management must be broad enough that the visions of the lower echelons of the organization fit within it.[3]

One segment of an organization's vision can be aimed at the consumer (for example, "Our vision is to have a fully staffed, high-quality, committed workforce that is efficient and effective in providing the highest quality service in our community"). Another portion can be directed at employees:

We envision an organization staffed by dedicated, enthusiastic, customer-oriented people who act as partners. Our people readily adapt to change, seek continuous technical improvements, and exhibit a caring attitude. Our organization is preferred by most patients and admitting physicians. It is the darling of third-party payers and a local preferred employer.

An organization's vision must be sustained through action consistent with the elements of the vision. Next, a vision is translated into an organizational mission that is then expressed in a mission statement. Goals are enunciated, strategy is developed, and action plans are constructed.

Mission

Mission statements proclaim the purpose of an organization or department, literally stating why this entity exists. Like visions, mission statements should serve to define the organization and inspire its employees. Too many supposed mission statements are vague, platitudinous, and quickly forgotten; most of them cannot pass the "snicker test" (the informal test that ought to be well understood by anyone who has ever reacted to a vague or hollow statement or motto as "corny" or "silly"). Too many organizations work hard to develop vision and mission statements, then let them become just framed pieces of paper decorating a wall.

An effective mission statement must be expressed clearly in a single, brief paragraph and in language that everyone can understand. When workers participate actively in the formulation of mission statements, they understand why the organization exists and what their work is all about. This understanding greatly increases the chances that they will do their best to make the virtual visions come to life.

Some mission statements include the vision plus goals and strategy. They answer the key questions of *why* ("Why does this organization or department exist?"), *what* ("What is our goal?"), and *how* ("How will we achieve our goal?"). What follows is a departmental mission statement appropriate for a small hospital unit. Note that it begins with a goal, adds objectives, and concludes with a strategy:

> We seek a service that surpasses the expectations of our clinician customers. We will improve the quality of reported results, shorten turnaround time, reduce costs, and promote a spirit of cooperation between our staff, our customers, vendors, and associates in other departments. To accomplish this we will meet weekly to analyze service needs, investigate complaints and suggestions, and explore new methods or equipment. We will make recommendations to management, monitor progress, and evaluate results.

Before accepting a mission statement, those responsible for managing the department or unit must ensure that it answers four critical questions:

1. Do you know where you want to be 5 years from now?
2. Is the mission clearly and definitely expressed in a single paragraph?

3. Is the statement expressed in language that a 10th grader can understand?
4. Will the mission be believable to everyone in the organization?

Goals and Objectives

Leaders share their visions and involve their associates in setting goals and objectives. Goals are characterized by specific ends or conclusions, whereas mission statements are generally open-ended. Many employees prefer activities leading to specific conclusions; for example, they usually prefer to work on projects rather than perform routine work because projects have clear destinations. All riders on a train know when they have arrived at the station. A significant number of retirees die shortly after retiring because mentally their goal—the end employment—has been reached and they have never developed a clear mission for dealing with the future.

Targets become more specific when goals are subdivided into objectives. Objectives are milestones to be passed on the journey toward reaching a goal. Objectives should be realistic, understandable, measurable, behavioral, achievable, and specific. An objective such as "reduce inventory costs" is not sufficiently specific. Instead, use "reduce inventory costs by 10% within 12 months"; any appropriate objective should relate *what* is to be done, *how* much is to be done, and by *when* it should be done.

Assign priorities to objectives and set target dates. Objectives should always be expressed in writing to provide a permanent record and to keep them foremost in the minds of employees. Although there should always be some degree of challenge—employees are motivated by achieving difficult but not impossible tasks—objectives must be attainable. If a plan holds little chance of success, it will frustrate rather than motivate. Here are some examples of over-inflated objectives:

- Within 12 months, a repeat survey of employee morale will show an increase in the average employee satisfaction rating from the current level 3 to level 2.
- By the end of the next quarter, we will provide point-of-care testing for all patients in the north wing.

Following are examples of objectives for a more comprehensive goal relating to customer satisfaction. Note that although these are open-ended, all are valid as ongoing objectives for this hypothetical organizational unit:

- Hire employees who are client oriented, technically or professionally competent, and likely to remain onboard.
- Provide an orientation and training program that stresses client satisfaction.
- Anticipate changes in customers' needs or expectations, and continually monitor customer satisfaction.

- Encourage all employees to participate in the planning and execution of new or improved services and in solving customer problems.
- Provide an intensive continuing education program that stresses client satisfaction.

Strategy

Successful organizations build on their existing strengths and eliminate their weaknesses or render them irrelevant. They constantly search for innovative ways to please their customers. The moves they make to please their customers, to position themselves relative to their markets, to adapt to the changing environment, and to address their relationships to their competition are reflections of their strategy. Keys to success in the pursuit of an organizational strategy include

- Vision, mission, goals, objectives, and action plans
- Committed and visible support of top management
- Effective and efficient systems, processes, and procedures
- Quality tools and techniques
- Sufficient time to carry out plans
- Empowered, caring, competent employees

Action Plans

Action plans are typically composed of five steps:

Step 1. Identify the Problem or Need

To identify and understand the problem or need, answer the following questions:

- Why is there a need for change? What is wrong with the present service or system?
- What are our strengths and weaknesses and those of our competitors?
- What are the potential gains, losses, or risks of a change?
- Who will be affected? What will it cost?
- What is likely to happen if no action is taken?

Step 2. Obtain and Analyze Data

Select a method of collecting information and build a databank. Be thorough when you collect information. Become familiar with statistical analysis and the use of charts, electronic data interchange, electronic mail, and workflow automation. Document current deficiencies and opportunities for improvement.

Step 3. Determine the Best Action

Appropriate action plans should answer the following questions:

- What is to be done?
- Why must it be done?
- When should it be started and when should it be completed?
- Who is to do it?
- Where is the action to take place?
- How should it be done?

Step 4. Carry Out the Plan

It is essential that a plan be doable, understandable, comprehensive, cost-effective, approved, and periodically reviewed. Complex plans should always include an executive summary describing how the proposal affects the mission statement and service quality and operating costs. Also to be added is your assessment of how you believe clients and employees will react to the changes wrought by the plan. The implementation process includes:

- Identifying resources (for example, people, supplies, equipment, facilities, time, and funds)
- Preparing checklists of important tasks to be performed
- Assigning tasks, authority, and responsibility
- Preparing work schedules
- Providing necessary training
- As necessary, formulating new policies, systems, and procedures

Sequencing and Scheduling of Tasks

Use Gantt charts, flowcharts, and flow diagrams or other logic diagrams to document tasks and analyze the times required for the work processes. On a chart, chronologically list the tasks to be done on one side opposite the appropriate calendar periods. See Chapter 9 for more information on charting.

Preparing a Budget

Estimate all costs associated with each task. Build in some slack for inflation or other unanticipated costs. Prepare a cost spreadsheet with tasks listed vertically and cost factors (for example, labor, supplies) listed horizontally and totaled at the right of each line.

Establishing Priorities

Priorities are a vital part of any plan. To avoid frustration, be flexible; that is, remain prepared to modify your priority list as circumstances change. Unexpected interruptions are the rule rather than the exception.

Step 5. Monitor the Process, Report Progress, and Make Adjustments

Formal control is planned control consisting of data gathering, analysis, and documentation. Informal control consists of day-by-day observations and impromptu meetings with other participants. Informal controls are more proactive than formal controls. Periodic status reports should be required for large projects.

Monitoring progress usually necessitates tying up some loose ends. These may involve changes in plans, reassignment of tasks, removal of barriers, or requests for additional resources. In all instances, the earlier a problem can be identified, the easier it is to correct.

Think About It

Conditions change, circumstances change, the environment is forever in a state of flux, so oftentimes plans are themselves not particularly useful. However, the planning process is invaluable.

Questions for Review and Discussion

1. If we believe that planning is so important, why, knowing this, do we so often rush directly into doing without pausing to plan?
2. What do we stand to gain from applying planning principles to supposedly routine activities?
3. What are two significant reasons why a particular objective or target may not be attained as planned?
4. What are the principal characteristics of planning that apparently cause many to bypass it altogether?
5. What kinds of plans are of most concern to the working supervisor? Why?
6. What are the primary differences between mission and vision?
7. What are the three essential components of an appropriate objective?
8. Assume the organization has a 5-year plan. When would formal planning again take place 5 years in the future? A year in the future? Some other time? Explain your answer.
9. What is the fundamental difference between goals and objectives?
10. Create an example of a sound objective to apply at the departmental level.

Exercise: Your Planning "Manual"

You are to write, preferably using full sentences but arranged in outline form, a departmental planning manual; that is, a guide for you and other supervisors to follow in preparing action plans for improving work methods, solving productivity problems, and addressing issues of quality. Be sure to provide for all of the required elements of an action plan.

Case: And Here We Go Once More

The position of business manager at Smalltown Hospital has been a hot seat, with incumbents changing frequently. When the position was vacated last May, the four senior employees in the department were interviewed. All were told that because they were at the top of grade and the compensation structure for new supervisors had not yet caught up with that of other positions, the position would involve just a miniscule increase in pay, an increment one could readily consider insultingly small. All four refused the position, and all were given the impression that they were not really considered qualified just yet but that they might be considered for supervision again at a later date.

That same month a new business manager was hired from the outside, and the four senior employees were instructed to show their new boss in detail how things worked in the department. Over the following several months the business manager's boss, the finance director, told all four senior employees that they had "come along very well" and would be considered for the manager's position should it again become vacant.

In October of that same year the manager resigned. However, none of the four senior employees got the job; the process was repeated, and again a new manager was hired from the outside.

Instructions

1. You are advised upfront to avoid allowing the most blatant errors and transgressions revealed in the case description to lead you to focus exclusively on the inappropriate management behavior. Rather, we are concerned here with operational planning. Viewing the department and its needs from the perspective of the finance director, describe how this shoot-from-the-hip manager, with appropriate forethought, could have properly planned for the department's supervisory transition.

2. Also, summarize what you believe to be the inappropriate consequences of the finance director's failure to plan.

REFERENCES

1. Dawson, R. 1992. *Secrets of power persuasion*. Englewood Cliffs, NJ: Prentice Hall, 277.
2. Hammer, M., and J. Champy. 1993. *Re-engineering the corporation*. New York, NY: Harper, 155.
3. Fisher, K. 1993. *Leading self-directed work teams: A guide to developing new team leadership*. New York, NY: McGraw-Hill, 136.

RECOMMENDED READING

J. G. Liebler and C. R. McConnell, *Management Principles for Health Professionals*, 5th ed., Chapter 4 "Planning," pp. 89–146 (Sudbury, MA: Jones and Bartlett Publishers, 2008).

Chapter 6

Team Leadership

*There are few, if any, jobs in which ability alone
is sufficient. Needed, also, are loyalty, sincerity,
enthusiasm, and team play.*

—William B. Given, Jr.

CHAPTER OBJECTIVES

- Define the kinds of teams to be found within the organization: those established for specific purposes, departmental teams, and the greater "team" unified by a common goal or directive.
- Enumerate both the benefits and the disadvantages of the use of special-purpose teams and examine their potential legal pitfalls.
- Establish the characteristics of an effective team.
- Examine the more common reasons for team failure.
- Describe the interactive forces involved in the formation, assembly, growth, and functioning of most teams, including team rituals and the relative strength of group norms and their role in a team's success or failure.
- Enumerate and discuss the responsibilities of team leadership and explore the implications of leadership style for effective team functioning.
- Suggest how the manager who inherits a team formed under a previous leader can constructively approach the new assignment.
- Briefly consider various means of evaluating and rewarding team performance, recognizing that most evaluation and reward systems focus on individuals, not groups.

As business enterprises of all kinds become more complex, they depend more on the effectiveness of group efforts and cross-functional activities. In health care, no longer do many individuals work as solo practitioners. For example, in the old days an emergency department (formerly referred to as an emergency room) was usually staffed by a physician and a few nurses and aides. Now an emergency department can feature dozens of professionals and technicians with diverse skills and experience who work as a team to save lives.

Various healthcare institutions are establishing satellite facilities, developing new services, implementing changes to comply with legal and other mandated requirements, and establishing comprehensive quality improvement programs. In the new healthcare paradigm, cross-functional teams regularly span departmental boundaries, and the third-party payers become senior partners in a healthcare team.

A team is a group of people who are committed to achieving common objectives. An effective team has members who work well together and enjoy doing so and who produce high-quality outcomes. Teams have become the utility vehicles of today's organizations.

The term "team" is actually representative of several different kinds of collectives, and it is necessary to know at most times the kind of team to which you may be referring. We regularly encounter special-purpose teams, departmental teams, and the greater team.

KINDS OF TEAMS

There are two types of special-purpose teams to be encountered in the workforce. One is characterized by the group that is assembled for a specific purpose, often including people from different departments or disciplines. This kind of team may be ad hoc, assembled for a one-time purpose and disbanded when that purpose has been served, or it may be ongoing with permanent or rotating membership and handling a certain kind of business or problem on a regular basis. These are the teams of team-oriented problem or quality circles, and these are teams such as your organization's safety committee or product evaluation committee chapter.

The departmental team is the group of employees and the single supervisor to whom they report. Team composition is simple; most people understand that everyone in the group has a job to do and together this accomplishes the work of the group. Such a group can operate as a number of individuals doing their jobs, but when these people are united into a true team the potential of the group is expanded dramatically. Much that is said about team building is applicable to forging and maintaining a strong departmental team, a collection of like-minded people who report to the same manager and cooperatively serve the common purpose of the department.

Frequent reference may be made to "the healthcare team," essentially all those involved in designing and delivering and paying for health care; this is the greater team. At times, the employing organization and all those it encompasses may be appropriately described as a team. Regardless of its kind, composition, reason for being, or degree of permanence, however, there is one significant factor that unites the members of any team: common purpose.

The Project or Employee Team

The organization of a project or employee team can be relatively simple: A decision is made to assemble a number of people with the appropriate knowledge, skills, or experience to undertake some specific task as a group. Most of these kinds of teams include both managers and rank-and-file employees, and because often nonsupervisory employees are the majority of team members, there are potential legal problems depending on the kinds of problems or issues addressed.

Just as important as leadership and cooperation are to the success of any team is sensitivity to potential legal pitfalls. Out of a desire to solicit employee participation, some organizations have discovered that a team can easily stray into questionable territory. There are areas of employee involvement in which teams are seen as intruding on the territory of labor unions, so there is a constant risk that a given employee team could be considered an illegal labor organization under the National Labor Relations Act, infringing on the rights of collective bargaining organizations.

An employee team or committee could be considered an employer-dominated illegal labor organization if the group gets involved in addressing any terms and conditions of employment such as with wages, hours, benefits, grievances, or such. A team might also be seen as an illegal labor organization if its recommendations result in management decisions but the group itself has no power to make the decisions.

Any team consisting of a majority of rank-and-file workers should have its activities strictly limited so that the group never addresses terms and condition of employment in any form. This essentially limits these kinds of teams to dealing with issues of quality and productivity.

BENEFITS OF TEAMS

Healthcare organizations regularly use teams to handle a wide variety of tasks and problems, taking advantage of the following benefits of teams:

- Greater total expertise. Although team formation is not a panacea, it does serve to refine a group's skills and expand its collective ability to solve problems. Teams are especially useful in addressing procedures, relationships, quality, productivity, and problem solving.
- Synergy. The total achievements of teams are invariably greater than what can be achieved by members acting independently.

- Improved morale. The motivational needs of affiliation, achievement, and control are satisfied in the team setting.
- Improved personnel retention. Employees are less prone to leave when they are members of teams, especially teams recognized for their successes.
- Increased flexibility. Team efforts reduce dependence on individuals. Services do not suffer when one member of a team is missing.

DISADVANTAGES OF TEAMS

Teams, however, have their downside. Healthcare managers must also be aware of the occasionally encountered disadvantages of team activity.

- Teams are not always needed. Many situations can be handled as well or better by individuals. Specialists handle specific situations more rapidly and without having to consult others or obtain the approval of other members of a work group. Attempts to introduce work teams in departments where there are no interdependencies are largely a waste of time and effort. However, in most healthcare departments, people do depend on one another.
- Team building requires start-up time. There is always that period early in the life of a team when effort must be invested in team formation but little if anything specific is being accomplished.
- Teams may become bureaucratic. A once-enthusiastic task force can become a self-perpetuating standing committee, and its business often becomes repetitious and boring.
- When fast action is required, someone—an individual—must take charge and get things rolling. When someone yells "fire," it is not the time to call a meeting.

CHARACTERISTICS OF EFFECTIVE TEAMS

An effective team can be described as follows:

- It is not always limited to a departmental work group or even an interdepartmental collection of members. As necessary, its members may include vendors, customers, people from other departments, and key support personnel.
- It possesses all the necessary knowledge, skill, and experience required to fulfill its charge and get the job done.
- As a body its members search for excellence in quality, productivity, and customer service. The team removes factors that inhibit quality performance.
- It welcomes innovation, new services, and improved processes and techniques.
- It is democratic. There is an absence of rank or formal authority. It has a leader who refers to his or her coworkers as associates, colleagues, or teammates, not as subordinates.

- It demonstrates effective multidirectional communication and as a group displays openness and candor.
- It remains inspired by a vision of what it is trying to accomplish. Its charge is clear, its goals are clear, and all members are unified in their pursuit.
- It actively constructs formal and informal networks that include people who aid in its mission.
- It possesses power based not on formal authority but on the credibility the team has earned through performance.
- Its members trust each other and are sensitive to each other's needs. They understand their roles, responsibilities, and degrees of authority.
- It addresses and eliminates conflict with other teams or nonteam employees through collaboration, coordination, and cooperation.
- It adheres to strict ethical and moral considerations.
- It conveys optimism, and its members have fun serving.

WHY TEAMS FAIL

There are many reasons why teams fail. Unrealistic mandates from higher management and a lack of purpose and direction are major factors. However, poor leadership is the most common problem leading to team failure. This may be the fault of the person to whom the team reports or the unwillingness of any individual team member to assume a leadership role. Reviews of failed teams almost always reveal a serious breakdown in communication.

Other factors also contribute to team failure:

- Domination of the team by players possessing higher status or greater knowledge or who are more aggressive. Other problem members include the pessimists, negativists, obstructionists, prima donnas, and goof-offs.
- Lack of organizational support, for example, insufficient resources or time, understaffing, or unpleasant work environments.
- Internal politics, hidden agendas, conformity pressures, favoritism, and excessive paperwork.
- The development within the team of cliques that have the effect of isolating the group from the rest of the organization.
- Destructive competition among team individuals for promotions, merit raises, recognition, and access to superiors.
- Unrealistic expectations, resulting in discouragement in the face of setbacks.
- Disapproval of a team's output or lack of action on the team's suggestions or recommendations by upper management. Also, failure of a team to respond to the ideas of its individual members can quickly quench enthusiasm.
- Lack of progress, failure to meet deadlines, setbacks, and bad results, any of which may be disheartening.

TEAM DYNAMICS

Team dynamics refers to the interactive forces brought to bear by individuals singly or collectively in a group activity. The success of group dynamics depends largely on how willing team leaders are to share authority, responsibility, information, and resources. Sharing is a large part of what participative management is all about.

Stages in Team Formation and Development

Stage 1: Confusion

This initial stage represents the transition from a group of individuals to a team. Participation is tentative or hesitant as members wonder what is expected of them. Team members may show suspicion, fear, and anxiety, and productivity may suffer.

Stage 2: Dissatisfaction

Some members may display negativity, hostility, bickering, or outright resistance. Infighting, defensiveness, and competition are common at this stage because a number of participants have not yet clearly seen themselves as members of a group. Low productivity may persist.

Stage 3: Resolution

If the team is to be successful, group norms and roles emerge once the dissatisfaction is on the way to resolution. Dissatisfaction and conflict diminish, and a sense of cohesiveness starts to develop. Dependence on strong formal leaders decreases. Cohesion is achieved when individual members feel responsible for the success of the team. Productivity attains moderate levels.

Stage 4: Maturation

Productivity is high and performance is smooth. Members have developed insight into personal and collective processes. Team members have learned how to resolve their differences and provide each other with constructive feedback. All of this requires time, and progress is not steady but up and down, in fits and starts. Mature teams experience some turnover in membership, mostly planned or expected. Moreover, priorities change, and a host of other variables constantly affect the nature and makeup of mature teams.

Group Norms

Group norms may be functional or dysfunctional. A functional form is evident when team members defend their team and their organization. A dysfunctional form develops when members believe their organization is taking advantage of them and they perhaps believe that teams are being assembled only to squeeze more work out of the participants.

In some dysfunctional forms, members struggle so hard to avoid conflict that team decisions suffer. Some conflict is essential to effective problem solving. Cohesion does not mean the complete absence of differences of opinion, arguments, or disagreements. Members of great teams can frequently be heard debating heatedly among themselves.

At the Marine Corps boot camp on Parris Island, drill instructors turn undisciplined men and women into confident leaders. Their group norms are high. The instructors teach a few key lessons and model the behavior they want:

- Tell the truth.
- Do your best, no matter how trivial the task.
- Choose the difficult right over the easy wrong.
- Look out for the group before you look out for yourself.
- Don't whine or make excuses.
- Judge others by their actions, not their race.
- Don't use "I" or "me."[1]

RITUALS AND STATUS SYMBOLS

Certain rituals are important to team success. The truly important positive rituals are mainly expressions of appreciation such as trophies, awards, parties, picnics, and special dinners. A negative ritual, largely undesirable but nevertheless a ritual of sorts, is the hazing or taunting of new employees. However, even some positive rituals may change their polarity; for example, the employee of the month award may be regarded with scorn when undeserving candidates are selected or deserving employees are overlooked.

Team status symbols can also be important. Take uniforms for instance. For years the long white hospital coat was worn only by attending physicians and senior house staff members. This is no longer the case; in many units the green scrub suit, complete with stethoscope, has become a uniform of choice of caregivers at all levels. The time-honored nurse's cap has all but disappeared, a sad passing in the view of the old-timers.

TEAM LEADERSHIP

> *A team is like a wheel in which each member*
> *is a spoke. It's the team leader's responsibility*
> *to have enough spokes and to keep*
> *the spokes the same length.*[2]

Many healthcare managers are unwilling or unable to adopt the concept of the self-directed team or even to take measures that encourage team efforts. Healthcare leaders must develop dual professional and supervisory skills. Team players must be given opportunities to develop their professional or technical skills (task skills) and skills that pull teams together. The five major responsibilities of team leaders are presented in detail as follows.

First, the team leader must plan. Team leaders must know how to make their teams effective and efficient, encouraging them to work smart. This cannot be accomplished without planning. Managers, in concert with their team members, should be able to answer these questions:

- What do our customers want or need?
- What additional information do we need?
- What past successes have we had in meeting the wants and needs of our customers?
- What are our strengths, and what needs to be improved?
- What new objectives and strategies do we need?
- How can we provide superior customer service faster or at less cost?
- What barriers do we face, and how can they be eliminated?
- Should we learn how others are doing what we are doing?

It is a team leader's job to develop people. Members of a work team, like members of an athletic team, have certain competencies, plus the ability to develop additional competencies. After structuring position descriptions and performance standards, a team leader selects the best people for the team and then orients, educates, trains, coaches, and motivates them. When a team is just getting started, ask all members to share a one-word characteristic each wants to see in a teammate and relate a scenario in which someone either possessed or lacked that trait. The story rounds out the understanding of the desired characteristic. If all members share a trait they value, the group will develop common ground on which to function.

Building a team is like converting a group of musicians into an orchestra. The leader must build the team. Team building involves developing relationships, communicating, holding meetings, and interacting on a daily basis. Leaders must create an atmosphere that supports and rewards creativity, openness, fairness, trust, mutual respect, and a commitment to safety and health. There must also be opportunities for career growth. Evaluate your team-building ability by taking the quiz in Exhibit 6–1.

The leader must truly lead the team. With the help of the other team members, team leaders prepare mission statements, set goals, develop strategies and plans, design or improve work processes, facilitate, coordinate, and troubleshoot. Lead-

Exhibit 6–1 Rate Yourself as a Team Builder

Check all of the following that you honestly believe describe you as a team leader.

____ My teammates help each other and share advice.

____ My team functions well when I am not present.

____ I hire people who may be able to perform some tasks better than I can.

____ I try to avoid hiring people who are just like me.

____ Each member of my team learns at least one new skill every year.

____ Each member of my team makes at least one suggestion every month.

____ I encourage both differences of opinion and suggestions for improvement.

____ We resolve rather than avoid conflict and problems.

____ Every member of my team can name all our external and internal customers.

____ Every member of my team can state the mission of our organization.

____ Every member of my team knows how our quality program affects our service.

____ Every member of my team follows safety procedures.

____ We prefer team over individual competition.

____ Every member of my team feels valued and accepted.

____ Our team has a can-do attitude. We strive to produce more than we promise.

____ Our team has a reputation for cooperating with other teams and individuals.

____ Our team attitude is one of optimism and enthusiasm. Negativism is rare.

ers must satisfy the affiliation needs of each team member. All employees want to be accepted by their colleagues. Leaders also encourage team members to train and coach each other.

The following is an example of a simple departmental mission statement:

Our department is committed to providing quality care at low cost to inpatients and outpatients. Staff members maintain their expertise through continuing education and development.

The leader must coordinate team activities. The team or its individual members often participate in cross-functional activities. Team leaders must coordinate these activities with other departments and services. Leaders must also be ready to serve as followers in some interdepartmental task forces, committees, and focus groups. Typical topics relate to new services, safety, quality management, customer satisfaction, and employee morale.

LEADERSHIP STYLE

The ideal leadership style for team building is based on the perception that personal power is having power *with* people, not *over* people. Situational leadership fits that perception. When new employees join a team, the leader uses a directive or paternalistic style; he or she tells the employees what to do, shows them how to do it, explains why the work is important, and relates how it fits into the big picture. Knowing that workers at this stage are frightened, insecure, and stressed, team leaders are patient and highly supportive at this time. Blanchard and Tager[3] warn against the "leave alone—zap" style in which inexperienced workers are not given enough direction and then are zapped when they make mistakes.

As employees develop confidence in their ability, the leaders back off, give them more latitude, and encourage them to solve their own problems. Some supervisors fail to move on from the initial show-and-tell stage to one that demonstrates confidence in their employees. The result is that employees remain dependent on their leaders or become annoyed with the continual spoon-feeding. Parents encounter the same difficulty when they continue to treat adolescents as though they were still small children. Most employees can advance to a comfortable level of self-confidence or even to a consultative stage in which they participate actively in planning, decision making, and problem solving.

The delegating style, in which team members assume some or many supervisory responsibilities, is appropriate for some team members. In this participative paradigm, the team leader serves as a facilitator and moderator rather than as a manager. Autonomous or self-directed teams feature a democratic system in which there are no supervisors or first-line managers. The team members select a group leader or leadership is rotated.

TAKING ON THE INHERITED TEAM

It is possible that you may be assigned to lead a new team, be promoted to a leadership role, or come into such a position as an outsider. If you have been a member of the team, you must make adjustments. If you worked previously with the group in a cross-functional activity, put aside old prejudices and stereotypes. Overlook previous areas of friction or irritation.

If you are new to the organization, get as much information as you can about the history, reputation, culture, and rituals of your new employer. Look into the leadership style of the previous group leader. How did the group members respond? How effective was that style? You can learn about this from the person to whom you report and from present team members. Hold group meetings to discuss mission, strategy, values, plans, your leadership style, and your previous experience.

Study the position descriptions for every job and the performance reviews of each employee, and hold individual meetings with team members. Find out as much as you can about their aspirations, complaints, and suggestions and about how you can make better use of their services. Prepare an inventory chart of the team's skills.

REWARDING TEAM PERFORMANCE

An increasing focus on teams necessitates changing the way organizations reward people. Traditional reward and recognition systems encourage individual achievement. When traditional merit pay systems are used, team cooperation often suffers. Individual rewards may cause competing employees to withhold information, undermine peers, and hamper cooperation. On the other hand, in the absence of individual rewards there is bound to be some resentment among the high performers, and the slackers have no incentive to improve. This dilemma is resolved by providing for both team and individual rewards. The group recognition builds camaraderie and cooperation. Also, when employees know their performance ratings are affected by the extent to which they display teamwork, the adverse effects of individual rewards are mitigated.

It is recommended that some of the following be included in your team reward strategy:

- Reward employees who participate in group functions such as serving on committees or working with problem-solving groups or task forces.
- Recognize the entire team when goals are met.
- Arrange for a team to present its special projects to other departments or to higher management.
- Bring in doughnuts or pizza for the team.
- Organize a car-wash day when managers wash employees' cars.
- Make special equipment or publications available.
- Thank the team at a special luncheon or coffee hour.
- Attend some of the team's committee meetings or problem-solving meetings. Comment favorably and encourage them to maintain their excellent performance.
- Display photos of the group in action.
- Broadcast congratulatory news about completed projects, new services, favorable customer comments, or successful cost cutting.
- Spruce up the lounge and provide amenities such as a coffeemaker and microwave oven.
- Take practical measures to improve communication systems, and make more information available.

- Eliminate unnecessary meetings and streamline necessary meetings to reduce wasted time.
- Delegate greater authority to the team.

Some of the foregoing suggestions initially appeared in the excellent book by Deeprose.[4]

Think About It

Although there has been much disparaging commentary about teams and committees and other such collectives, few if any forces in business are as potentially creative and productive as a team of honest, fully participating individuals who are united in pursuit of a common objective.

Questions for Review and Discussion

1. What do you believe should be done concerning a team member who monopolizes every meeting? What if the person who is monopolizes is the team leader?
2. Why is shared authority important to proper team functioning?
3. Fully explain why some conflict is essential to effective team problem solving.
4. Many times we have heard that "A camel is a horse designed by a committee." Why have so many committees and teams inspired such cynical descriptions?
5. What do you believe is the primary hazard or significant drawback of a permanent team?
6. What is the "situational leadership" mentioned in the discussion of leadership style? Explain.
7. If you have just inherited a team and must take over today as its leader, how would you go about quickly getting an understanding of the style of the previous leader?
8. How would you suggest that a generally well-functioning team handle a single nonproductive member?
9. What are two significant disadvantages of team action? How can these disadvantages be overcome?
10. What do you believe is meant by the claim that team power is based on credibility? How do a team and its leader go about acquiring this power?

Case: The Quiet Bunch

You learned during your first week on the job as the newly hired admitting supervisor that each departmental supervisor was expected to lead one of the hospital's numerous quality improvement teams. It came as no surprise that the team to which you were assigned was the team your predecessor, the former admitting supervisor, had served as leader. Your team, you soon learned, consisted of several of your department's people plus employees from a scattering of other departments.

As you held individual meetings to become acquainted with both your Admitting employees and other members of your team, you were quickly inundated with complaints and other indications of discontent from both Admitting employees and quality team members. There were vocal complaints about the way the department had been run and complaints about the "useless quality improvement team." From a couple of the employees who served both in Admitting and on the quality team, you received complaints about "those who shall remain nameless" who regularly "carry tales to administration."

You listened to all the complaints. You detected some common themes in what you were hearing, leading you to believe that perhaps some misunderstandings could be cleared up if some of the issues could be aired openly with each concerned group. You scheduled two meetings, one for your Admitting staff and one for the quality improvement team. You felt encouraged because a number of individuals had told you they would be happy to speak up at such a meeting.

Your first meeting, held with the Admitting staff, was brief; nobody spoke up, even when urged to do so in the most nonthreatening way possible. Your subsequent meeting with the quality team was no better. You got zero discussion going with either group, although before and between the meetings you had been bombarded by complaints from individuals. This left you extremely frustrated because most of the complaints you heard were group issues, not individual problems.

Questions

1. What can you do to get either or both groups to open up in a group setting about what is bothering them?
2. Can you suggest what might lie in the immediate past that could have rendered these employees unwilling to speak up?
3. Because you have two groups (with overlapping membership) to be concerned with, where would you initially concentrate your efforts?
4. What might you do concerning the charges that someone is "carrying tales to administration?"

Case: The Weekly Team Meeting

Fourteen people from perhaps seven departments make up the long-standing methods improvement team that you were assigned to take over as leader 3 months ago. It has been the practice to hold a meeting at 3:00 p.m. every second Wednesday, or perhaps we should say you attempt to hold it at 3:00

because about half of the team members are more than 5 minutes late, and two or three are usually late by 15 minutes or longer. You have found also that roughly half of the group has not completed assignments they were given at previous meetings.

You have made repeated announcements about being there on time, but to no avail. Come the alternate Wednesday at 3:00 p.m., you usually find yourself and the same few punctual members present and waiting for the latecomers.

Questions

1. What can you do to encourage punctuality at the team meetings?
2. How do you suggest addressing the problem presented by the team members who do not complete their assignments?

REFERENCES

1. Ricks, T. E. 1997. What we can learn from them: Lessons from Parris Island. *Parade Magazine* November 9:4–6.
2. Keye Productivity Center. 1991. *How to build a better work team*, 2nd ed. Kansas City, MO: Keye Productivity Center, 3.
3. Blanchard, M., and M. A. Tager. 1985. *Working well: Managing for health and high performance*. New York, NY: Simon & Schuster, 50.
4. Deeprose, D. 1994. *How to recognize and reward employees*. New York, NY: AMACOM, 100.

RECOMMENDED READING AND LISTENING

D. Harrington-Mackin, *The Team Building Tool Kit* (New York, NY: AMACOM, 1994).

T. A. Kayser, *Mining Group Gold: How to Cash in on the Collaborative Brain Power of a Group* (El Segundo, CA: Serif Publishing, 1990).

A. R. Montebello, *Work Teams That Work* (Minneapolis, MN: Best Sellers Publishers, 1994).

M. Sanborn, *Team Building: How to Motivate and Manage People*, 2 audiotapes (Boulder, CO: CareerTrack Publishers, 1989).

W. Umiker, *The Empowered Laboratory Team: A Survival Kit for Supervisors, Team Leaders, and Team Professionals* (Chicago, IL: ASCP Press, 1997).

R. S. Wellins, W. C. Byham, and J. M. Wilson, *Empowered Teams: Creating Self-Directed Work Groups that Improve Quality, Productivity, and Participation* (San Francisco, CA: Jossey-Bass Publishers, 1991).

Chapter 7

Leaders and Managers

*Leadership involves remembering past mistakes,
an analysis of today's achievements, and a
well-grounded imagination in visualizing
the problems of the future.*

—Stanley C. Allyn

CHAPTER OBJECTIVES

- Explore the relationship between leadership and the culture of the organization in terms of how one has an influence in shaping the other.
- Describe the perceived differences between the popular conceptions of "leading" and "managing."
- Identify the principal characteristics defining the various styles of leadership.
- Identify several special leadership approaches that some leaders have incorporated into their approaches to managing people.
- Discuss some of the primary activities of leadership at the department level that are pursued in the process of getting things done through people.
- Examine in detail the characteristics of effective leaders applicable at all levels of organizational activity and in all organizational settings.
- Identify a number of the more common mistakes made by supervisors in attempting to fulfill their leadership responsibilities.

Leadership is not a process learned in seminars by remembering and following a specific number of steps or behaving according to some formula. Rather, leadership is either intuitive or gained through experience. The best leaders strive to develop the leadership skills of their teammates so that the success of the team

155

does not depend on a single person. Many organizations have failed because charismatic leaders did not develop new leaders, and when they were no longer around their backups were unable to step up and perform as required.

True leaders can influence people over whom they have no formal authority. This is often referred to as "horizontal management," and it is one of the marks of a true leader. To meet today's interdepartmental needs for coordination and cooperation, healthcare managers must possess leadership ability.

The best leaders understand how their own prejudices influence the way they lead. Because they can confront their own prejudices and shortcomings, they can deal with those of others. They censure intolerance and ensure equality of opportunity. They pay special attention to people outside the mainstream culture, knowing that these people can easily come to feel isolated. They learn about the values and cultural heritage of others and become aware of the differences in communication styles and interpersonal relationships.[1]

If you are a full-time manager, you are rewarded for what your employees do and for the responsibilities you fulfill, not for the tasks you perform personally.

ORGANIZATIONAL CULTURE

Management provides

- Mission statements (why we do what we do)
- Visions (what it will look like when we get where we want to go)
- Goals (so we know we have arrived)
- Strategies (the journey taken in getting there)
- Values (how we behave on the journey)

Leaders shape the culture of their organization, and to a considerable extent the culture shapes the leaders. Organizational culture can be defined as follows: a "pattern of basic assumptions that has worked well enough to be considered valid and to be taught to new members as the correct way to perceive, think and feel in relation to coping with problems."[2] and "A culture in which the leadership style of the manager features coercion and other direct power processes is less effective than a culture characterized by collaboration and participation."[3] In other words, organizational culture is simply the broad-based perception of the way things are done at work.

The healthcare culture of today demands pervasive and honest communication: openness and authentic interaction in all operations. This translates into the sharing of knowledge, skills, news, experiences, problems, and setbacks. The result is learning at all levels.

To foster a service-oriented culture, supervisors express values that are spin-offs from the mission statement. They put values into action by treating employees as they want customers to be treated. They get personally involved in service activities, and they use periodic meetings of their work groups to inspire and solve problems.

LEADING VERSUS MANAGING

To address apparent differences between leading and managing it is necessary to get beyond dictionary definitions and examine popular perceptions. The definitions in any good dictionary tell us that leading and managing are essentially the same, often to the point of defining one in terms of the other. And any thesaurus we might care to open lists "leader" and "manager" as synonyms for each other. In terms of word meanings on paper, leader and manager are one. When we speak of differentiating between leader and manager, however, we are dealing not with word definitions but with human perceptions. A great many people perceive a difference between the two words, and in the mind of the perceiver, perception is reality.

Decide for yourself how much difference, if any, exists between the two terms. When you hear about leadership do you equate this with management? Or do you perceive a difference between the two, with leadership somehow the more acceptable, indeed the more desirable, of the two? Popular perception generally holds that leadership is on a somewhat higher level than management, and it is this perceived difference on which most of what is said here about leadership is based.

The foregoing enables us to say that we have among us many good managers but that we often experience a shortage of good leaders. Business schools develop managers, not leaders, although, unfortunately, some schools readily attach the label of leader to their graduates. Perception, plus observation of such individuals in action, suggests the following differences between leading and managing:

- People obey managers because they must or they expect to; people follow leaders because they want to.
- Leaders envision (for example, Martin Luther King, Jr.'s "I Have a Dream"); managers marshal resources to achieve the visions of others.
- Leaders often rely on their intuition. Although some managers are intuitive, managers by and large rely more on analysis, objectivity, and rationality.
- Leaders generally demonstrate more self-confidence and are willing to take more and greater risks than managers.
- Leaders stress creativity; managers are more likely to stress conformity.
- Managers project power over people; leaders project power with people.
- Managers strive to satisfy the needs and wants of their customers; leaders endeavor to astonish customers by exceeding their wants and needs.
- The goals of managers usually arise from necessity; the goals of leaders are more likely to arise from desire.

- Managers are more like scientists (methodical, organized); leaders are more like artists (spontaneous, creative).
- Managers say, "I will support you"; leaders say, "Follow me."
- Managers are more concerned with the how; leaders are more concerned with the what.
- Managers seek obedience; leaders seek commitment.
- Managers control; leaders empower.
- Managers correct problems; leaders prevent problems.
- Managers learn how successful people do things and emulate them; leaders explore new paths.
- Managers may place primary emphasis on system, structure, and process; leaders are more likely to emphasize team building and personnel development.

There have been long-standing discussions concerning whether management is an art or a science; the conclusions drawn usually suggest that it is both art and science. We might further suggest that if indeed there is a real fundamental difference between management and leadership, it is that management is more science than art whereas leadership is more art than science.

Certainly, managers can be leaders as well. It is most likely that the very best managers are also excellent leaders.

BASIC LEADERSHIP STYLES

Clusters of particular leadership characteristics and behaviors have been described as leadership styles. Like clothing styles, leadership styles come and go; some even return for a while, and others prevail for a time and vanish, never to return.

Authoritarian Leadership

Leaders who use this style are often described as task oriented, paternalistic, or autocratic. They "run a tight ship," and they order or direct their employees. This style is also referred to as top-down or "I" (the leader comes first) management (also referred to as Theory X).

Authoritarian leaders believe that people must be controlled closely and provided with external motivation (for example, pay, benefits, and good working conditions). They are task oriented rather than people oriented. They tell employees what they want but do not necessarily tell them why. They do not invite input from their people and may in fact even discourage input. Autocratic leaders encourage dependency. Employees of authoritarian leaders often exhibit apathy or hostility.

A subset of the pure authoritarian style is the paternalistic approach. Paternalistic managers exhibit either the features of a kind, nurturing parent—call this the benevolent dictator—or those of a critical and oppressive parent or, if you will, a tyrant. A paternalistic approach is appropriate when one is dealing with emergencies in which one must instantly obey without questioning (for example, fire or disaster) and may at times be the best way to deal with inexperienced or insecure employees or hostile people who challenge authority.

"Micromanagement" is a form of authoritarian leadership. Despite nearly universal condemnation of the practice, many supervisors micromanage because they believe their employees are unable to function without them. They believe they must stay on top of things at all times to prevent mistakes or to make sure the work gets done. They are certain their staffers are incapable of making decisions. Some simply believe this is what managers are supposed to do. To be successful in the long run, however, these managers must learn to delegate authority and trust their employees.

Participative Leadership

Leaders who behave according to this style are often referred to as people oriented. They run a "happy ship." This style is also described as bottom-up or "we" (all of us together) management (Theory Y).

Participative leaders believe that people want to work and are willing to assume responsibility. They believe that, if treated properly, people can be trusted and will put forth their best efforts. Participative leaders motivate by means of internal factors (for example, task satisfaction, self-esteem, recognition, and praise). They explain why things must be done, listen to what employees have to say, and respect their opinions. They delegate wisely and effectively.

There are several subsets of this style. When in a consultative mode, leaders seek input from their followers before making important decisions. When in a delegative mode, leaders share responsibility with their colleagues.

One simple way to learn whether participative management is in place is to keep track of the number of suggestions each employee makes annually. In many Japanese companies, where participative management flourishes, each employee submits dozens of ideas each year. Equally important is the percentage of suggestions that are acted on by management.

Participative managers can be counted on to articulate two magic phrases: "What do you think?" and "I need your help."

Theory Z Leadership

Unrelated to Theory X and Theory Y, Theory Z was labeled as such primarily to distinguish it from authoritarian leadership. Originated by the Japanese, Theory Z is characterized by employee participation and egalitarianism. It features guaranteed employment, maximum employee input, and strong reliance on team mechanisms such as quality circles.

Bureaucratic Leadership

Terms descriptive of this style include rules oriented, by-the-book management, and "they" management (essentially impersonal). Bureaucratic managers act as monitors or police. They enforce policies, rules, procedures, and orders from upper management. They tend to be buck-passers who take little or no responsibility for directives and who often experience near-paralysis of thought and action when encountering a situation for which no rule exists.

For the most part bureaucrats do not see themselves as bureaucrats. The very term bureaucrat conveys a negative connotation, and few if any people will consciously label themselves that way. Nevertheless, bureaucrats exist in some places in large numbers, and they often play negative, self-serving political games. They advance in stable or static organizations by not making mistakes, reducing risk taking, and blaming others. Government agencies and military services tend to house many bureaucrats, as do occasional other organizations such as major not-for-profits in which employees have found the maximum likelihood of continued employment and minimum likelihood of significant change.

True leadership is incompatible with the stifling character of bureaucracy. However, a bureaucratic style may sometimes be suitable for operations in which tasks must always be performed in the same way (for example, sorting mail or typing reports).

Situational Leadership

Terms used to describe this style include contingency based, flexible, adaptive, and "different strokes for different folks" leadership. As the name suggests, flexible leaders adapt their approach to specific situations and to the particular needs of different members of the team. As employees gain experience and confidence, the leadership style changes from highly directive to supportive (from task related to people related). For example, two new employees may start work on the same date. If one has had previous experience and the other has had none, different directive styles are needed. A show-and-tell approach is required by the novice, but the same may not be appropriate for the experienced person.

A practical guideline is to consider a consultative or delegative style in reference to areas of expertise and to provide specific direction in areas of weakness. Some managers, in an effort to always be participative, fail to be directive when direction is needed.

Laissez-Faire Leadership

This kind of leadership is described as hands off, fence-straddling, absentee, Catch-22, and "not me" management. Laissez-faire managers avoid giving orders, solving problems, or making decisions. They are physically evasive and are sometimes nowhere to be found when needed. Verbally, they are often masters of double-talk.

A positive form of laissez-faire leadership is the democratic style. Presently in vogue, it features self-directed (autonomous) teams in which leadership is delegated to highly trained work groups. The members of these teams know more about the organization and are better trained, more motivated, and more productive than their counterparts in traditional settings. They solve problems, redesign work processes, set standards and goals, select and monitor new employees, and evaluate team and individual performance.

Clearly, this hands-off style of leadership can work extremely well if sufficient leadership has been involved in building the teams and seeing that they are properly charged and appropriately oriented. However, this can also be the refuge of the lazy or incompetent manager who is self-deluded into believing that he or she is backed by strong self-directed teams when this is nowhere near the case.

LEADERSHIP APPROACHES: SPECIAL VARIATIONS

Manipulation

Unfortunately, organizational management includes its share of manipulators. Manipulative managers get people to do their bidding by

- Intimidating them, in effect making them fearful of the consequences of not complying
- Engaging in emotionalism: using anger, tears, yelling, or playing to seek sympathy
- Making people feel guilty if they do not immediately do what is wanted of them
- Implying the employees owe them something for past favors
- Name dropping; for example, "The Director will be very unhappy if this isn't resolved right away" (more or less intimidation-by-proxy)

Management by Crisis

Management by crisis is also referred to as "fire-fighting management," and it is always easy to recognize the people who use this approach. They are surrounded by noise, confusion, and emotional upheavals. Every day is characterized by a series of crises for them. They complain that they cannot get things done because they are too busy putting out fires. They react rather than anticipate; they solve problems instead of preventing them. Their behavior suggests that planning is a concept completely foreign to them. Everything they do is reactive; they are never proactive.

Management by Exception

Managers who have adopted the practice of managing by exception act as facilitators, supporters, and resource people. Their message is "I do not interfere as long as your actions and results remain within broad limits of acceptable performance. Come to me with problems you can't solve or when you need something I can get you." Management by exception is appropriate when leading certain categories of professionals or specialists.

Management by Objectives

Management by objectives is considered by many to have been one of the management "flavor of the month" ideas that enjoy immense popularity for a while and then fade away. This particular approach probably remained popular longer than most other special management approaches. Throughout the 1960s and beyond many firms established management by objectives programs. True, it has lost much of its popularity, but a number of its basic features remain useful. For example, when you are reviewing the performance of an employee, one helpful way to focus on the future is to do so in terms of future performance objectives.

Management by Wandering Around

This particular informal practice involves little more than its name implies. At its heart, however, is something of great importance to managers at all levels: visibility. A manager who is "out there" to see and be seen accomplishes much more than the manager who never leaves the office.

CONTEMPORARY LEADERSHIP ACTIVITIES

Leadership has evolved over the ages, and at different periods of time the emphasis has been on different leadership activities. The needs of the times influence the activities in which the leaders of any era are engaged. For example, given the state of health care today, today's leaders are more likely to be concerned with matters of productivity and cost containment than were the leaders of 30 or 40 years ago. For the most part contemporary leaders are deeply involved in the following activities:

- Team building and group problem solving
- Cross-training for efficiency and flexibility
- Employee empowerment
- Improved quality and customer service
- Cost cutting
- Managing change (new services, products, or facilities)
- Staff reductions or other personnel rearrangements
- Decentralizing activities or establishing satellite activities
- Worker safety and health programs
- Environmental preservation
- Patient home care
- Point-of-care services (for example, expanded bedside services)

FOUNDATION OF LEADERSHIP

One prominent feature of a well-led work force is the absence of cynicism. Cynicism disappears when employees respect their leaders. They respect their leaders because they perceive them as competent, caring, truthful, and ethical. Those leaders "walk the talk." Their behavior matches their words, and it features integrity and trust. Trust has two parts: being trusting (that is, displaying the ability to believe in others) and being trustworthy (that is, fully deserving others' belief in them). Leadership in its strongest form is leadership by example. Leading is not only walking the talk, it is also talking the walk. Talking the walk is explaining to your employees why you are taking or rejecting certain actions. Your employees must respect what you do and understand why you are doing it. If you achieve that with your employees, you will succeed as a leader.

CHARACTERISTICS OF EFFECTIVE LEADERS

Leaders must be walking mission statements who make their visions come alive by talking about them with enthusiasm and conviction. They must express themselves in attitudes and actions more than in words. Enthusiasm is almost magical; it is a positive and optimistic mindset that generates energy, enhances creativity, builds networks, and attracts other winners. It is especially necessary for the supervisory functions of motivation, communication, delegation, and problem solving.

No matter how you feel, start the day with a burst of enthusiasm. ("Fake it 'til you make it.") Throughout the day, feed positive thoughts into your subconscious mind by saying positive things about your performance. Surround yourself with other optimistic doers. Shun the complaining observers. If you hang around with turkeys, you will never soar with the eagles. Use success imagery; that is, visualize good outcomes in whatever you do. Recharge your energy by relaxing or meditating, especially after setbacks.

Good team leaders use both the helicopter approach and the management-by-wandering-around approach. Like helicopters, they hover over the work area where they can view the total operation. When they spot trouble, they descend for a closer look or to get involved. In the proactive management-by-wandering-around process, leaders do not wait for people to bring problems into their offices. Instead, they make frequent visits to each workstation. Here they spot potential problems and ask for suggestions. They also seek ideas from vendors and customers.

As evident from the following lists, a number of factors figure into the characteristics of an effective leader. It should perhaps be conceded at the outset that only rarely will a particular leader possess every last one of the following characteristics. It is, in fact, possible to point to any number of apparently successful leaders who are clearly lacking several of what we might consider essential characteristics. However, every leader who has succeeded in the job has enjoyed one significant advantage: the followers accepted that person's leadership.

Important Characteristics of Effective Team Leaders

- Effective team leaders are competent.
  - They possess both professional and team leadership skills, recognizing that the leader must be proficient in both sides of the role.
  - People look up to them and respect their expertise.
  - Their opinions and advice are sought after by associates both inside and outside their departments.
  - They are asked to serve on important committees.
  - They work to constantly improve their professional and leadership capabilities.
  - They can answer most questions, and when they cannot answer they know where to get the answers.
  - They cooperate fully with their counterparts in other departments.
- Effective team leaders are emotionally stable.
  - They exhibit a relaxed leadership style.
  - They remain cool and calm under trying circumstances.
  - They handle stress well.
  - When they get upset with people, they focus on behavior, not on personalities or individual traits.
- Effective team leaders get the job done.
  - They provide a sense of direction and set high expectations and standards.
  - They expect and demand good performance.
  - They are well organized and always prepared.

- They are proactive; they anticipate and prepare for change.
- They focus on important matters; they do not nitpick.
- They place the right people in the right jobs.
- They do not waste their time or that of their followers.
- They stimulate innovativeness and invite ideas.
- They provide all the resources their teams need.
- They get rid of the deadwood.
- Effective team leaders are effective communicators.
- They use memos, meetings, and other communication channels effectively.
  - They provide clear instructions and request feedback to make sure that their directions are understood.
  - They are articulate and persuasive, but they do not manipulate people.
  - They are excellent listeners and are easy to talk with.
  - They share information but do not repeat gossip.
  - They do not withhold bad news, but they deliver it with consideration.
  - They are effective teachers.
  - They provide feedback, both positive and negative, as needed.
  - They criticize behavior, not people or personalities.
  - They are quick to praise and to give credit. They praise in public and criticize in private.
  - They acknowledge their own mistakes and make sure they learn from them.
  - They always seem to know what's going on.
- Effective team leaders are unafraid.
  - They thrive on responsibility.
  - They take risks, and they bend rules when doing so makes sense.
  - They are innovative and flexible.
  - They chalk up failures to experience.
  - They keep their fears to themselves.
  - They encourage creativity and risk taking.
  - They accept responsibility for failures.
- Effective team leaders are credible.
  - They are dedicated to telling the truth.
  - They keep their promises and fulfill their commitments.
  - They admit their mistakes.
  - They do not take credit for the ideas of others.
  - They do not play favorites, and their credibility is above reproach.
- Effective team leaders develop committed followers.
  - They care about their followers, and they show it.
  - They are willing to roll up their sleeves and help out when necessary.
  - They go to bat for their people.
  - They empower employees and encourage autonomy and self-reliance.

- They provide their people with whatever they need to get their work done.
- They allow people freedom in how the work is done, but they insist on getting the results they expect.
- They do not play favorites.
- They are fully as attentive to people below them as to those above them in the organization, perhaps even more so.
- They invite and respect the opinions and suggestions of all their employees.
- They provide opportunities for employees to use newly learned skills or previously untapped skills.
- They encourage and support suggestions, comments, and proposals from all management levels.
- They articulate what they value and back this up with their everyday behavior.
- They reward cooperation as highly as they reward individual achievement.
- They are helpful and anticipate the needs and problems of their team members.
- They defend their people from outside harassment.
- Effective team leaders exhibit charisma.
  - They maintain a childlike fascination with things and people.
  - They make it a point to catch people doing something right . . . and tell them so.
  - They hold a warm handshake and smile for a few seconds longer than the other person.
  - They use the other person's name often during conversation.
  - They project energy and enthusiasm.
  - They are good role models.

COMMON SUPERVISORY MISTAKES

Everyone makes mistakes; to do so is human nature. But when someone in a leadership capacity makes a mistake the effect is frequently multiplied through the leader's area of responsibility. A mistake by a supervisor is often visible throughout the immediate work group and beyond. Supervisory errors diminish the effectiveness of the supervisor and, even more so, often negatively affect the effectiveness of the group. Here are some of the more common mistakes made by supervisors:

- They pass the buck and try to avoid accepting accountability, which is directly contrary to what is expected of a supervisor.
- They fail to delegate properly and empower their employees, leaving themselves open to overwork, criticism, and burnout while the employees go unchallenged.

- They take the narrow view of customer service and ignore their internal customers.
- They pay inadequate attention to budgetary concerns and fail to control costs.
- They associate with losers, mindless of the effect on their credibility.
- They use a cookie-cutter approach to managing, as though every problem was solvable by formula.
- They seek to be liked by all instead of seeking respect.
- They tolerate incompetence and fail to set performance standards.
- They neglect their own training and career development as well as the training and development of their employees.
- They recognize and reward only their top performers.

Exhibit 7–1 The 12 Commandments of Leadership

1. Know what you want.	7. Let your expertise show.
2. Take control of your career.	8. Rely on others.
3. Believe in yourself.	9. Look for opportunities.
4. Go for the goal.	10. Learn the ropes.
5. Enjoy the game.	11. Never stop networking.
6. Be capable.	12. Get a mentor.

Think About It

As for the best leaders, the people do not notice their existence. The next best, the people honor and praise. The next the people fear; and the next, the people hate. When the best leader's work is done, the people say, "We did it ourselves!"

—Lao-tzu

Questions for Review and Discussion

1. Explain what is meant by the following statement: "Leadership cannot be taught, but it can be learned."
2. How is it that true leaders can often influence people over whom they have no formal authority?
3. How does a successful, well-functioning, self-directed leaderless team get to be that way? Does it ever need a leader once it achieves that state?
4. A portion of the chapter addressed perceived differences between the terms "manager" and "leader." What, if any, do you believe are the differences between "manager" and "boss"?

5. Under what kind of leadership would an organization be least likely to change? Why do you believe this is so?
6. The quotation from Lao-tzu cited earlier states that "When the best leader's work is done, the people say, 'We did it ourselves!'" Do you agree with this? Why or why not?
7. Why is failure to delegate thoroughly and properly of particular importance to a group's leader? Provide several possible reasons.
8. As a supervisor, what do you believe you would have to do to become comfortable with managing by exception?
9. Why do you believe teams and team building have enjoyed such increasing popularity in recent years?
10. Why do we claim that leading by example is extremely important? What are some of the problems that can arise when we fail to do so?

Essay: Examining the Micromanager

Surely most, if not all, readers of these pages are familiar with the term "micromanagement." Perhaps some have found themselves in circumstances in which they have been micro-managed and thus have gained some firsthand understanding of it. Micromanagers often give employees the distinct impression that they do not trust them or think them capable of correctly fulfilling their responsibilities on their own.

In essay form, explain in detail why you believe micromanagers behave as they do and why supervisors who attempt to lead by micromanaging employees are destined for failure in the long run.

Case: That's Her Responsibility, Not Mine

Susan Wilson is the administrative supervisor of Diagnostic Imaging (formerly the radiology department) at Central Hospital. Supervising in an expanding department and coping with steadily increasing outpatient activity, she found her workload increasing to the extent that she believed help was required with some of her duties. Taking a hard look at tasks she could legitimately delegate, that is, tasks that did not require supervisory authority, she settled on her monthly statistical report. The report itself was fairly easy to create, but gathering the necessary data consumed a fair amount of time.

She selected employee George Peters to do the report and provided him with all necessary instructions, even to the point of creating a detailed written procedure. She believed George was capable of doing a thorough job; he had sufficient time available to incorporate the report into his workload, and she further thought that George might appreciate some variety in his work. George expressed no feelings for nor against doing the report.

A few days after assigning the report Susan discovered that the current report had not yet been started and that if it were not completed at once it would be late. Susan reminded George; his reply was that other necessary work was delaying the data collection. Susan emphasized the need to get the report done on time, but George seemed in no particular hurry to get into the task.

The following day Susan accidentally overheard a portion of a conversation between George and another employee to whom George was saying: ". . . her lousy statistics. I think she should keep doing it herself. After all, that report's her responsibility, not mine."

Instructions

1. Identify and describe any actions Susan might have taken incorrectly in delegating the statistical report to George.
2. Decide what, if anything, Susan can do to try to correct the attitude revealed by George in his comments to the other employee.

REFERENCES

1. Rosen, R. H. 1996. *Leading people*. New York: Viking Press, 207, 213.
2. Schein, E. 1990. Organizational culture. *American Psychologist* 45:109–119.
3. Young, J. A., and B. Smith. 1988. Organizational change and the HR professional. *Personnel* 65:44.

RECOMMENDED READING

A. M. Barker, D. T. Sullivan, and M. J. Emery, *Leadership Competencies for Clinical Managers: The Renaissance of Transformational Leadership* (Sudbury, MA: Jones and Bartlett Publishers, 2006).
K. Blanchard and S. Johnson, *The One-Minute Manager* (New York: Berkeley Publishers, 1982).
K. Blanchard and R. Lorber, *Putting the One-Minute Manager to Work* (New York: William Morrow and Company, 1984).
T. Kent et al., "Leadership in the Formation of New Health Care Environment." *Health Care Supervisor* 15, no. 2 (1996): 27–34.
R. S. Kindler, *Managing the Technical Professional* (Menlo Park, CA: Crisp Publishers, 1993).
R. H. Rosen, *Leading People* (New York: Viking Press, 1996).
S. A. Stumpf, "Strategic Management Skills: What They Are and Why They Are Needed." *Clinical Laboratory Management Review* 10, no. 3 (1996): 231–44.

Chapter 8

Budgets and Cost Control

A budget is a practical means of telling
the money where to go—
rather than simply wondering
where it went.

—Anonymous

CHAPTER OBJECTIVES

- Introduce the concepts of budgets and budgeting, and establish their essential role in the operation of an organization or organizational unit.
- Identify the significant functions and elements of budgets, and enumerate the principles and rules of budgeting as they apply to the supervisor.
- Introduce the controlling process as related to budgets.
- Identify overtime as a sometimes significant cost element, and suggest steps for keeping overtime under control.
- Describe a number of significant cost-reducing measures, including rightsizing and reengineering, that the supervisor may encounter when it becomes necessary for the organization to bring expenses down into line with revenue.
- Identify the role of benchmarking in cost control.

The cost-containment measures imposed on healthcare providers have greatly increased the importance of cost control. Supervisors are key people in the control and reduction of expenses. Essential parts of the supervisory role are participating in the preparation of departmental budgets, suggesting cost-cutting measures, and directing the application of control measures.

171

BUDGETS AND THEIR FUNCTIONS

Planning

The preparation of a budget is part of the planning function. A budget is itself a plan, a financial plan for the conduct of business in the near future. A budget provides a financial map of coming activities. It also contains information vital to the potential determination of new charges and adjustments to various costs of doing business. Budget planning normally starts at executive levels and trickles down to first-line managers. It should coincide with the review of major policies and the reassessment of plans and goals.

Controlling

> *A tight budget brings out the best creative
> instincts . . . . Put him under some financial
> pressure. He will scream in anguish. Then he'll
> come up with a plan that, to his own amazement,
> is not only less expensive, but is also faster and
> better than his original proposal.*
>
> —Robert Townsend[1]

The administration of a budget is part of the controlling function, and the budget itself is the most powerful tool available for controlling. A budget creates a greater awareness of costs on the part of employees, and it also helps them achieve goals within stated cost expenditures.

The finance department usually provides supervisors with weekly or monthly cost reports of expenditures against budget. These reports highlight variances that serve as red flags for remedial action.

Evaluating

Performance appraisals of supervisors usually include the assessment of how accurately they forecast their expenses and how well their expenditures match the monies allocated. Variances can reflect poorly on a supervisor's financial skills unless the deviations result from factors not under his or her control. Staying under budget is not always a cause for celebration. Having funds left over at the end of the year might sometimes indicate efficient management of resources, but it can just as readily result from careless budgeting.

Principles and Rules of Budgeting

- Expenses must always be charged to the department or cost center that incurs the expenditures.
- Every item of expense must be under the control of someone in the organization.
- Supervisors and managers responsible for complying with expense budgets must participate in budget preparation.
- Supervisors must not be held responsible for expenditures over which they have no control.
- Unused budgeted funds may not be carried over from one annual budget to the next.
- Unused funds for capital expenditures may not be transferred to operating expenses or vice versa.
- Requisitions for individual expenditures require approval by some authority.
- "Slush funds" or contingency funds not specifically identified are not permitted, but supervisors should try to allocate some monies for unexpected needs.

Revenue

Depending on the budgeting approach of a particular organization, revenue figures may come from the finance or information services departments. Computerized billing makes it possible to calculate revenue for each department or section and to use these figures to project anticipated future revenue.

Most supervisors are usually not directly accountable for revenues, but they can be helpful in determining charges for the services that their departments render. Without the supervisors' cost data, finance departments have no legitimate basis for figuring out charges or for forecasting profit or loss. In predicting revenue and costs, it is necessary to consider not only historical growth trends but also changes in the anticipated workload because of the introduction of new services, procedures, or equipment.

Preparation of Budgets

A breakdown of expenses charged to a department by categories, such as salaries, benefits, and supplies, is essential (Table 8–1). Expenses should be recorded on an ongoing basis.

A budget cannot be adequately prepared the week before it is due. To prepare an itemization of expenses, collect expense figures for several months. Annualize the figures by dividing the year-to-date expenses by the number of months recorded, then multiply by 12.[2]

Table 8–1 Example of a Forecast Budget: Chemistry Section

Item	Annual Expense ($)
Medical/surgical supplies	300
Employee welfare	20,640
Pension	2,112
Postage, freight, express	408
Salaries and wages	281,572
Departmental supplies	367,800
Quality control	28,667
Travel	672
Publications	100
Education	336
Repairs and maintenance	12,000
Total Direct Expense	714,607

During the year suggestions or proposals may turn up that involve additional expense or cost-cutting opportunities. Record all these. Take into account increases in supply expenses, service contracts, and continuing education expenses when planning a forecast budget.

Capital Equipment

Usually, a separate budget or a section of the overall budget is set aside for capital equipment. Many organizations project their capital equipment budgets out for 2, 3, 4, or 5 years into the future. This extended capital budget may change from year to year as priorities change and unforeseen circumstances arise, but more often than not capital funds are strictly limited organization-wide, and what one department might want in the short run may have to defer to something another department critically needs. Supervisors who must be knowledgeable of rates of obsolescence of major pieces of equipment often seek this kind of information from manufacturers or suppliers.

Replacement items and new equipment are among the most expensive budgetary items for some cost centers (for example, laboratory or radiology services, where single pieces of equipment can run into the hundreds of thousands of dollars). The capital equipment budget should reflect the costs of these items.

Wages, Benefits, and Overhead

The figures for salaries, benefits, and overhead are not budgeted by the operating departments. These numbers come from elsewhere, primarily from the finance department. However, other areas may be involved; for example, budgeted benefits costs may come from the human resources department. This is appropriate because supervisors have no control over these items and cannot be held responsible for them.

Salaries represent more than 60% of operating expenses for most cost centers in the typical healthcare organization. Therefore when administrators want to cut costs the first area they scrutinize is usually personnel expenses. It is essential to keep detailed records to justify work hours and overtime and make certain that the figures going into the budget are as accurate as possible.

Management is ordinarily unwilling to approve requests for additional staff, even when there is a projected increase in the workload, unless the need can be proven on paper. Reports of crises that have occurred because of personnel shortages can help in the justification process. This also holds true for equipment problems and requests for new apparatus.

CONTROLLING PROCESS

Always be prepared to defend the budget figures you submit. With or without modifications by higher management, the budget revisits supervisors at least monthly in the form of a responsibility summary (Table 8–2). This simplified report shows actual expenditures compared with budgeted amounts for the month. The full report received by the supervisor also shows cumulative actual and budget figures for the year to date, so it is possible to track performance against budget in cumulative fashion throughout the year. Variances are shown for each budget category. When variances exceed a certain amount, supervisors generally must submit an explanation.

Review these reports soon after receiving them. If an item is not clear or may be in error, seek clarification from finance or information services, whichever division issues the report. Be prepared to discuss the variances with your immediate superior.

CONTINUING CONTROL OF OVERTIME

One area in which supervisors can have a significant effect on a department's cost picture is the control of overtime. Overtime is an organizational necessity that is misused or abused as often as it is applied correctly. As an element of labor cost it is sometimes seen as an extra expense to be avoided by all means, yet there are

Table 8–2 Responsibility Summary

Current Month	Actual	Budget	Variance
Inpatient revenue	160,414	167,081	6,667*
Outpatient revenue	106,591	78,129	28,462
Total patient revenue	267,005	245,210	21,795
Medical/surgical supplies	207	25	182*
Employee welfare	2,299	1,663	636*
Pension	1,059	1,059	0
Postage, freight, express	31	34	3
Salaries and wages	25,166	23,263	1,903*
Departmental supplies	43,788	30,650	13,138*
Quality control	211	211*	0
Travel	118	118	0
Publications	59	59	0
Education	49	1,000	951
Repairs and maintenance	72,810	57,871	14,939*
Total direct expense	267,005	245,210	21,795
Total patient revenue	72,810	57,871	14,939*
Direct expense			
Operating gain or loss	194,195	187,339	6,856

*Unfavorable variances (i.e., low revenue or high expenditures).

times when overtime is the best response to a particular need. The determination and payment of overtime are dictated by provisions of the Fair Labor Standards Act, the federal wage and hour legislation that governs a number of aspects of employment. Overtime is often taken for granted, and it can readily get out of control. It is the task of the department supervisor to maintain control of overtime, adhering to a budget and taking active steps to ensure that only essential overtime is approved and worked.

- Overtime is viewed and applied in a number of ways. As suggested, it is often used to correct mistakes, and as certainly implied above it is used to compensate for inefficiencies and time wasted. However, it is used primarily, at least in intent, to accomplish necessary, or perhaps unanticipated, work when there is more work to be accomplished within a given time period and too little regularly scheduled staff available to get it done.

- Overtime is a constant concern for a great many working healthcare supervisors. There are almost always needs arising, and the nature of a healthcare operation dictates that coverage be present. In some health organizations functions that cannot be done today can be left until tomorrow, but a great many necessary tasks cannot wait until the next day.

- Some overtime is essential and absolutely unavoidable. Some, however, is questionable and perhaps optional, and some is unnecessary and completely avoidable. All overtime, even to some extent that which is essential, is controllable. And the strongest point of control is the first-line supervisor, the immediate supervisor of the people who work the overtime.

- The continuing emphasis on the need for cost containment undoubtedly increases the pressure on supervisors to control overtime and to economically justify all overtime used. Certainly, the department that uses too much overtime—and "too much" can be difficult to define—will have cost problems. However, there may also be a problem in a department that seems never to use overtime; it is highly probable that such a department is overstaffed.

Causes of Overtime

The causes of overtime are many and varied, but within the organization that may be experiencing excessive overtime these causes often include all or most of the following:

- Variations in workload: unexpected changes in demand, unanticipated changes deadlines, and genuine emergency situations
- Absenteeism: demonstrable, direct relationship between employee absenteeism and the need for overtime
- Tolerance of substandard performance
- General acceptance of overtime as a normal practice rather than an exception
- Lack of supervisor accountability (for example, if the supervisor does not have to answer for overtime use, it becomes accepted as normal and less likely seen as a recourse for handling true exceptions)
- Rigid scheduling practices
- Bargaining unit work rules stating that only certain classifications of employees can perform certain kinds of work
- Inappropriate or insufficient equipment and inefficient physical work area

At its worst continuing overtime is costly, disruptive, and counterproductive. Even at its best continuing overtime becomes part of the employee's supposedly "normal" time available for doing work and the work tends to spread over that available time.

Toward Control of Overtime

There are several general approaches available for the control of overtime.

- Regulate demand. In some departments it is possible to take actions that regulate the demand on the department's services. The approaches available for the regulation of demand include working on a reservation or appointment basis, promoting low-demand periods, and using complementary scheduling. In general, any steps that can be taken to regulate demand serve to decrease the need for overtime.
- Analyze and improve staffing practices. Possibilities include cross-training employees; using floats as appropriate; using per diem, casual, or optional staff; increasing hours of some of the department's part-time employees; and constantly reevaluating scheduling practices.
- Analyze and improve work methods. Ineffective work methods and procedures and inappropriate equipment and workplace layout all tend to depress productivity and increase the pressure for overtime.
- Control absenteeism. To address absenteeism directly is to directly address the problem of excess overtime as well.
- Manage responsibly. Consider yourself accountable for the level of overtime usage in the department.

CUTTING COSTS

When there is a severe financial crunch, organizations take multiple remedial measures. When drastic action is not imperative, managers introduce changes one at a time to observe the effects of each change before undertaking the next measure.

Cost control involves more than cutting staff and working more efficiently. It can also involve improving inventory control and seeking price relief from suppliers. Reductions of salary, overtime expenses, and benefits may be necessary but are often counterproductive if made prematurely or without examining their full implications.

Typical hospital responses are the laboratory responses reported by Jahn.[3] These included freezing or limiting expenditures for filling vacancies, capital spending, salary increases, and cutbacks in continuing education. If these were not sufficiently effective, layoffs would follow.

Rightsizing

Rightsizing is matching staffing to workloads to become more efficient. It differs from downsizing, which is simply laying off people in response to declining business or to save money, although more often than not the terms are used interchangeably, along with several other labels for adjusting the size of the work force. Restructuring, acquisitions, mergers, and financial reverses all frequently result in reductions in force. Employers can accomplish reductions in force through early retirements, attrition, hiring freezes, voluntary separations, or reduced work hours. These measures are often insufficient, however; thus involuntary separations are exercised as the last resort.

The best time to begin this process is before financial constraints demand major staff reductions. The first step for executives is to analyze the workload and find out what can be done to reduce it without decreasing services or turnaround times. The second step is process reengineering or restructuring.[4]

Chief executive officers must decide whether to base furloughing on seniority or on a person's value to the organization. If the latter, supervisors play an important—and often painful—role in the selection process. Also, it is extremely important that whatever scheme is used for determining staff reductions is applied consistently throughout the organization and in a completely nondiscriminatory manner and that documentation exists to support the rationale for selecting those who are to be laid off.

Responses to the Call for Reduced Personnel Costs

Initially, you should try to determine whether you can increase efficiency or reduce costs by transferring or merging activities within your organizational unit. If you must transfer tasks from professional or highly trained technical employees to less educated workers, insist that the latter be trained first or that they are closely supervised until they have the work fully under control. Tap into the observations and recommendations of the persons who do the work. They have practical ideas on how workflows can be streamlined. When workers participate in the planning, they are less likely to object to changes, even when the changes involve staff reductions.

If the mandate calls for reduction of payroll to a certain level, hold brainstorming sessions with your employees. Get their ideas for reducing salary costs without laying people off. Some senior people may decide that this is a good time for them to end their careers. Some full-time employees may opt for part-time employment, and part-timers may be willing to reduce their hours, especially if they have more schedule options.

Handling Those Who Leave

Supervisors must face the anger of those who leave and the apprehension of those who remain. The reaction of some people who are laid off is often much like that of patients when they are told they have cancer. First, there is disbelief, then anger or depression, and finally acceptance. Be tolerant of their anger, bitterness, and hostility, and be empathetic when the tears flow. Console yourself with the knowledge that most of these people will recover and find new and sometimes more satisfying positions. Answer their questions honestly, and make sure they get the information they need about benefits and eligibility for unemployment benefits.

If outplacement services are available, encourage employees to take full advantage of them. These may include placement services, help with job applications and interview techniques, psychological testing, and training for new vocations. Use your personal network to try to find new jobs for them or at least to steer them in the right direction. Do not hold out false hopes for recalls. If the likelihood of rehire is high, keep in touch with them.

Handling Those Who Remain

Layoff survivors often feel guilty and depressed because of losing friends and colleagues. They may experience a drop in self-esteem and morale. In the back of their minds is the fear of future layoffs. Remain visible. Do not hide in meetings or bury yourself in paperwork. Share their concern about their friends who are laid off.

Distance yourself from idle gossip, but keep yourself informed. Share that information. Explain the rationale for the changes. Answer questions honestly, and listen to expressions of frustration and fear. Do not wait for staff meetings or newsletters to keep your team informed. Call special meetings whenever you acquire new information.

You and your staff must pick up the slack. Ask for the participation and cooperation of your staff in closing ranks and getting the job done with fewer people. Point out the increased need for teamwork and for everyone to make a special effort. Prepare a list of duties and responsibilities that others must assume. Announce assignment changes, and provide any additional training that may be needed. Use your reward and recognition system to reward your team or individuals who make special efforts.

Process Reengineering

Reengineering may prove to be the most cost-effective mechanism in healthcare institutions. Without reengineering, cost-reduction initiatives achieve only modest results. The major savings will not come from departmental reengineering but from those initiatives that address interdepartmental functions and that break down compartmentalization. These include abandoning obsolete systems, forming cross-functional, self-directed teams, amalgamating jobs, discarding old rules and assumptions, introducing new technologies, and creating new principles for task orientation.

BENCHMARKING

Benchmarking is the search for best or preferred practices and is accomplished by comparing current systems or processes with highly successful ones. Your goal is to increase efficiency, cut costs, or improve service. The comparisons may be with standards reported in the literature or with observations at the facilities of recognized leaders. Benchmarking usually leads to some form of process, system, or structural reengineering. It is an essential tool in cost control and quality improvement with improved patient and fiscal outcomes at stake.

A benchmarking strategy usually requires data searches, networking, and creation of cross-functional teams. When national standards are unavailable, your external networks can be crucial to establishing standards. Questionnaires and other survey tools are often used to locate the best benchmark sources.

The usual approach consists of (1) a data-collection phase that may include literature searches or site visits, (2) an analysis phase, and (3) an action plan. The planning process may involve use of flowcharts and other problem-solving tools; it is frequently necessary to dissect workflows to find problems or weaknesses.

Kreider and Walsh[5] reported a highly successful benchmarking project that ensured decreased ventilator-associated pneumonia and intensive care unit costs. With a cost-restructuring plan based on benchmark information, one hospital reduced its operating budget by $33 million dollars.[6] Rotondi et al.[7] benchmarked their preoperative patient routing system. After they identified causes for variation, they created multidisciplinary improvement teams to improve the pinpointed areas. Mitchell[8] found that the national benchmark for turnaround time between surgical cases was 13.5 minutes, whereas his hospital's time was 19.9 minutes. A quality improvement team carried out solutions that produced an 18% improvement. The cost–benefit analysis showed a potential revenue enhancement of about $300,000.

Think About It

The best defense against having to make painful reductions at crunch time is to have your unit's cost picture under control at all times. Control consists of more than just monthly budget reports to review. The information comparing budgets with actual expenditures is important, but it is only part of the equation. True cost control is information plus action.

Questions for Review and Discussion

1. Often, the productivity of a work group decreases after a layoff, even though there is more work to be done overall. Why might this be so?
2. In budgeting, why are funds for operating expenses and funds for capital expenditures always kept separated?
3. Describe one set of circumstances under which a supervisor may be largely powerless to affect a particular expense charged to the department.
4. Is overtime expense fully controllable, partially controllable, or not at all controllable by the supervisor? Explain.
5. If the numbers say the organization has to reduce 20 positions, and 20 employees leave via resignation and retirement, why might it still be necessary to reduce positions further and even engage in some hiring?
6. How can benchmarking assist the supervisor in determining whether a staff reduction may be necessary?
7. What conditions or circumstances in your own department should you consider before deciding to reduce staff?
8. The term "reengineering" literally means "engineering again." Why is so much so-called reengineering not true reengineering?
9. As a department supervisor, why might you often not get what you have asked for in the capital budget?
10. What information can the department supervisor often supply to finance or information services that can help in developing revenue projections?

Case: Let's Jettison the Deadwood

Two supervisors, Robert and Janet, were in charge of sections of the building services department of Central Hospital. They had a fairly close working relationship; they were in a position to cover for each other on occasion and usually did so successfully. Overall, however, they had quite different styles of dealing with their employees.

The long-anticipated word came down that declining admissions and sharp cuts in reimbursement rates necessitated staff reductions. Robert's staff would have to be reduced by three people; Janet's staff was projected to lose two people. On Monday they learned officially of the impending cuts; they had to have names turned in by Wednesday, and layoffs would actually occur Friday. Monday afternoon they found themselves discussing the layoffs.

Robert said, "How is this supposed to be done? I missed the meeting with the boss this morning thanks to a toxic material spill. I got the information secondhand, and all I know is that I've got to dump three people."

"Right," Janet replied. "And I have to lose two. These are the times when I'm almost sorry I took a supervisory job."

"Why? Employees come and go. This just means a few have to go unwillingly. I figure on taking advantage of this to jettison some deadwood."

"How can you do that? You weren't there this morning—it was pretty strongly indicated we should go by seniority. You know, last in, first out. Unless there's some compelling reason to the contrary."

"Compelling reasons I've got lots of," Robert responded. "One of mine who's going is the last in, no trouble there. But the other two are major pains I've wanted to get rid of for a long time."

"Got lots of documentation?"

"Who needs it?" Robert tapped the side of his head. "It's here. Overall I'll be getting rid of the three worst producers in the group. Nobody will have any idea how people are picked for layoff, and, anyway, at least two of these bozos should already figure they're on the way out."

Questions

1. Is Robert justified in wanting to get rid of "the three worst producers in the group"? Under what circumstances might he be able to do this without creating another kind of problem?
2. What is the possible exposure to the organization and to Robert if he were to go ahead and "jettison the deadwood" as planned?
3. What can you infer from the case about the supervisory styles of both Robert and Janet?

Exercise: The Budgeting Game

There are two common methods for approaching budgeting at the department level. With the more sensible approach, the department supervisor carefully determines the funds needed for each of the group's controllable budget categories and submits as accurate a budget as possible.

The second method, and unfortunately one that is used a great deal of the time—perhaps even most of the time—requires involvement in "the budgeting game." In this approach the supervisor calculates an honest budget, then tacks on an additional percentage to each budget category on the assumption that higher management or at least the finance department will assume a certain amount of padding and arbitrarily reduce each category by some unknown percentage. The essence of the "game" lies in being more accurate than the other party in guessing the percentage of padding and thus the percentage of reduction. This sometimes goes back and forth for three or four iterations until the department's total lands where higher management or finance wants it to be.

Instructions

In essay form you are to comment on the validity of the budgeting game, but, most important, you are to describe how you as an individual supervisor might be able to break out of the "game" and submit an honest, accurate, and acceptable budget.

REFERENCES

1. Townsend, R. 1971. *Up the organization.* New York: Fawcett, 173.
2. Sattler, J. 1980. *Financial management of the clinical laboratory.* Oradell, NJ: Medical Economics, 124.
3. Jahn, M. 1995. Laboratorians speak out on benefits, managed care, and the bottom line. *Medical Laboratory Observer* 27(5):29–33.
4. Medvescek, P. 1997. Rightsizing the right way. *Medical Laboratory Observer* 29(7):102–106.
5. Kreider, C., and B. A. Walsh. 1997. Benchmarking for a competitive edge. *Medical Laboratory Observer Supplement* (September 1997):S26–S29.
6. Cohen, E., and E. Anderson-Miles. 1997. Benchmarking: A management tool for academic medical centers. *Best Practical Benchmarking in Healthcare* 1(2):57–61.
7. Rotondi, A. J. et al. 1997. Benchmarking the perioperative process. 1. Patient routing systems: A method for continual improvement of patient flow and resource utilization. *Journal of Clinical Anesthesia* 9(3):159–169.
8. Mitchell, L. 1997. Benchmarking, benchmarks, or best practices? Applying quality improvement principles to decrease surgical turnaround time. *Best Practical Benchmarking in Healthcare* 1(2):70–74.

Chapter 9

Decision Making and Problem Solving

Nothing is impossible: there are ways which lead to everything; and if we had sufficient will we should always have sufficient means.

—Francois de La Rochefoucauld

CHAPTER OBJECTIVES

- Establish the importance of decision making in today's work organizations and outline its implications for the role of the supervisor.
- Present a generalized process for logically approaching and solving large or complex problems.
- Introduce a number of tools that are useful in problem-solving activities.
- Explore the intuitive process and its key role in problem solving.
- Briefly explore the role and potential usefulness of group problem-solving activities.

Problems are inevitable when people work together. The hallmark of a well-managed team is not the absence of problems but whether the team resolves problems effectively. Many managers continue to blame their employees for most of the problems that occur, but all too often the real villains are faulty management decisions.

DECISION MAKING TODAY

The rate of organizational, technical, legal, and operational change constantly increases. Many of the decisions related to these changes have great impact on financial stability or job security, role alterations, assignments, and customer satisfaction.

Today's supervisors are forced to make decisions that were less common previously, decisions related, for example, to downsizing, reassigning, cross-training, and replacing professional employees with less qualified personnel. Also, critical shortages of certain specialists demand quick hiring decisions before competitors snap up these scarce resources.

Our society has grown increasingly litigious. Flawed decisions lead to legal nightmares, for example, harassment and discrimination complaints. Employee safety, satisfaction, and ethical issues are becoming more numerous and complex.

People-related decisions are by far the most important to the individual supervisor. Hiring, training, disciplining, promoting, and discharging employees all demand careful consideration.

DECISION MAKING AND LEADERSHIP

Autocratic leaders make decisions without soliciting input from others. Consultative leaders get input from others before deciding. Democratic leaders participate with their staffs in making decisions, and delegative leaders turn the process over to others.

Higher management deals chiefly with decisions that relate to major outcomes or long-range strategies, the *what* of running the organization. Supervisors deal principally with operational processes, how day-to-day operations are conducted.

When to Avoid Making Decisions

Every situation needs to be considered in light of one simple question: is a decision really necessary? Avoid making a decision when

- The apparent difficulty is not your problem (others will take care of their own problems).
- The problem is likely to correct itself, or interference is likely to make matters worse (in other words, if it ain't broke, don't fix it).
- You or others are emotionally upset or there are serious attention distractions.
- More information or advice is needed before an informed decision can be made.
- The problem is one that should be delegated. Most decisions should be made at the lowest possible organizational level—as close to the scene of action as possible—as long as those delegated to do so are capable and willing.

Essential Trinity for Effective Decisions

An effective decision must be

- The most cogent decision.
- Timely as to when it is made and when it is implemented. Professionals often procrastinate because they are looking for more additional data; they fall prey to "paralysis from analysis."
- Acceptable to the people affected. Many managers are adept at making decisions but fail to persuade people to carry them out.

Dual Cognitive Functions

There are two cognitive approaches to decision making and problem solving: analytical and intuitive. Analytical, or left-brain function, provides rational, logical, scientific thinking. Intuitive cognition, or right-brain function, provides creativity and inspiration.

Left-brain thinking is essentially a flowchart process. Analytical people rely on algorithmic processes, plans, reports, computer printouts, and step-by-step procedures. They exercise judgment at each step and exclude anything that is irrelevant. Managers and investigators who treat problem solving as a science often fail to come up with creative ideas because they depend entirely on this rational approach. Managers tend to use more left-brain thinking and more effective leaders rely to a great extent on their intuition.

Intuitive thinking depends on data buried in our unconscious minds, which are like computers with almost unlimited memory storage capability. Unfortunately, what we file in these cerebral banks may be difficult to recall; it can be like trying to access a computer program for which we have lost the password. Unlike computer-stored data, brain information is constantly and unconsciously analyzed, synthesized, and reformatted.

Innovative people possess deeper insight or experience stronger gut reactions. They visualize more than their rational counterparts. They prefer diagrams to printouts. They often throw logic out the window. An intuitive thought process can seldom be flowcharted; rather, it is hop, skip, and jump.

> Common sense is a combination of logic and intuition, the left and right brain working in tandem.

Coping with Many Minor Problems

Supervisors face innumerable little problems and decisions every day. Much of the time solving problems is the most important responsibility of the supervisor. If there were no problems, we might need no supervisors. Their subordinates bring problems into their offices by the carload. Better training, planning, coaching, delegating, and policymaking work wonders in cutting down on the number of these daily interruptions.

The Stop-Look-Listen Approach

Approach these daily questions or problems like you approach a railroad crossing:

- Stop what you are doing.
- Look interested.
- Listen carefully.

If the problem remains unclear, ask pertinent questions. Then ask those who bring you the problems what they believe should be done. Much of the time they will have thought through their problems and may have better solutions than you can offer on the spur of the moment. If you agree, approve their suggestions and congratulate them. If they keep bringing in the same problem, tell them that they do not need your decision every time.

Tell your people that you expect them to practice completed staff work. Explain to them that the military term, completed staff work, means that a staff member who comes in with a problem must also bring in ideas on how best to solve the problem and perhaps also a recommendation as to which possible solution may be best. Participative management requires much completed staff work.

If the problem is one that only you can solve, provide your answer on the spot or get back to them without undue delay. Follow up when appropriate.

THE LOGICAL PROCESS: KEY STEPS IN SOLVING LARGE PROBLEMS

Step 1. Prepare a problem statement. Diagnosis is often the most important part of problem solving, but it is often the most neglected part. Too often, people offer solutions before they really understand the problem. Poor problem statements can lead people astray. For example, the problem statement "Lack of clear policy relating to sick leave" is not likely to lead to solving a problem of excessive absenteeism that exists because of poor enforcement by the supervisor.

Step 2. Obtain and interpret the facts or data by asking the following questions:

- When was the problem first noted?
- How serious is it?
- Is it getting better or worse?
- Is it more complicated than it first appeared? In what way?
- What is the cause? (This is the most important question.)
- How was this handled in the past? What were the results?

Step 3. Generate alternatives (as many as possible).

Step 4. Formulate criteria to evaluate the alternatives. There are two types of criteria. Absolute criteria must be satisfied by an acceptable solution (for example, "No increase in costs or personnel"). Differential criteria are used to compare and contrast the various alternatives (for example, turnaround time, schedule convenience, availability of supplies, and degree of expertise required).

Step 5. Evaluate the alternatives and select the best one.

Step 6. Look for flaws in the choice. Ask many "what ifs." Avoid the jigsaw puzzle fallacy. The jigsaw fallacy is based on the false assumption that there is only one good solution (for example, a jigsaw puzzle must have four straight edges). Often there are several equally satisfactory solutions: The edges of life's puzzles are seldom straight lines.

Step 7. Develop an action plan.

Step 8. Carry out the plan. If there is hesitation about implementing the plan, ask what would be the worst possible thing that could happen if the plan was carried out. Also ask what the worst possible thing would be if you do not take the risk.

Step 9. Follow up. If what you are doing is not working well, make the needed changes.

USEFUL TOOLS FOR PROBLEM SOLVING

Bar graphs (Figure 9–1a) display a series of numbers (for example, the number of patient visits on each day of the month). When a bar graph shows the distribution of a variance, it is called a histogram (Figure 9–1b). *Pareto diagrams* (Figure 9–1c) display the frequency of occurrences listed in order of importance or frequency. A *scattergram* (Figure 9–1d) shows the correlation between two variables. *Run charts* (Figure 9–1e) plot data over time. They exhibit trends, cycles, or other patterns in a process (for example, attendance records, turnover, or customer complaints). *Control charts* (Figure 9–1f) illustrate values that are either in control or out of control. In Figure 9–1f, the solid horizontal line represents an average or normal value. The spaces between the solid line and the dotted lines are acceptable values, usually plus or minus two or three standard deviations. Any value outside the dotted lines is an out-of-control value.

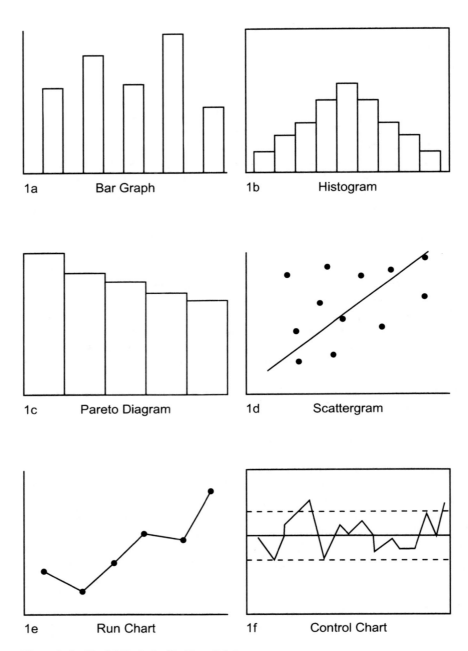

Figure 9–1   Useful Tools for Problem Solving

A *flow chart* (Figure 9–2a) represents a series of steps or events arranged chronologically. *Cause and effect diagrams*, also known as fishbone diagrams, are useful in an early stage of problem solving or when one is considering potential problems (Figure 9–2b). A cause and effect diagram forces a focus on potential causes. On each leg (each bone), possible factors are recorded and grouped according to different categories (e.g., process, human, equipment, or policies). *Pie charts* (Figure 9–2c) illustrate relative numbers or percentages. *Gaussian curve charts* have bell-shaped curves that show frequency distributions. These are among the most common quality control charts (Figure 9–2d). *Force field charts* are useful when considering the advantages and disadvantages of a new service, process, procedure, or piece of equipment. The opposing considerations can be illustrated and quantified by a force field chart (Figure 9–2e).[1] *Checklists* (Figure 9–2f) are used as reminders or for documentation of activities. Shopping lists, daily "to do" schedules, and validation of records are just a few uses for this ubiquitous tool. Figure 9–2f is a partial list of tests that a new laboratory technician must be qualified to do.

The *Gantt chart* (Figure 9–3) is a graph with activities listed on the vertical axis and time units on the horizontal axis.[2] It is used to find the shortest total time required to reach a goal by showing how much time each activity requires and which activities can and cannot be done simultaneously. In Figure 9–3, note the overlapping of several activities.

Program evaluation and review technique (PERT) charts (Figure 9–4) were developed to reduce and control the time required for large projects. The PERT chart is composed of activities and events. On the chart, events are represented by circles. Arrows show the time necessary to complete events. When there are steps carried out simultaneously, different times are needed for each of these parallel steps. In Figure 9–4, the lines could represent the following steps:

A–B   time for a request to reach a workstation
B–C   time for blood collection and delivery to a laboratory
C–D   time for serological testing
D–E   time for immunohematological testing
E–F   time for delivery of blood product to patient

The critical path represents the sum of the times for individual steps in the path that require the most time. In Figure 9–4, the critical path is A-B-C-D-F because it takes longer to do the serological tests than to do the routine compatibility tests.

The *break-even chart* is a scatter diagram (or scattergram) in which the Procedures and the Expenses—variable and fixed—are plotted with diagonal lines representing total revenues and total costs (Figure 9–5). The point at which the diagonal lines cross represents the financial break-even point. The number of procedures performed below that crossing shows a loss; those above that crossing show a profit.

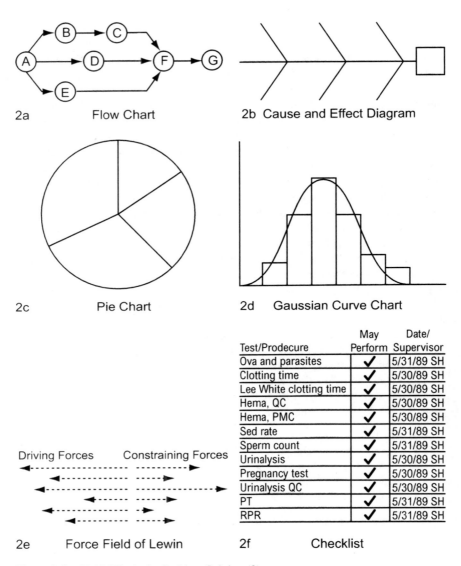

2a   Flow Chart   2b Cause and Effect Diagram

2c   Pie Chart   2d   Gaussian Curve Chart

Test/Prodecure	May Perform	Date/ Supervisor
Ova and parasites	✓	5/31/89 SH
Clotting time	✓	5/30/89 SH
Lee White clotting time	✓	5/30/89 SH
Hema, QC	✓	5/30/89 SH
Hema, PMC	✓	5/30/89 SH
Sed rate	✓	5/31/89 SH
Sperm count	✓	5/31/89 SH
Urinalysis	✓	5/30/89 SH
Pregnancy test	✓	5/30/89 SH
Urinalysis QC	✓	5/30/89 SH
PT	✓	5/31/89 SH
RPR	✓	5/31/89 SH

Driving Forces   Constraining Forces

2e   Force Field of Lewin   2f   Checklist

Figure 9–2   Useful Tools for Problem Solving (2)

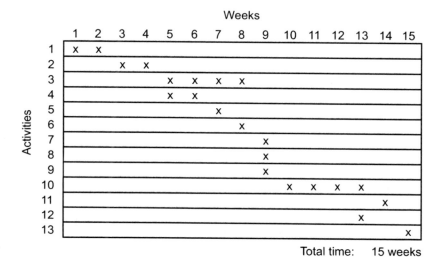

Figure 9–3   Gantt Chart

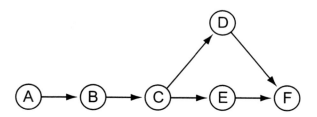

Figure 9–4   PERT Chart with Critical Path

Likert charts (Figure 9–6) are useful when one is comparing and contrasting multiple factors of performance at two different times (e.g., before and after a change).[3]

Computer Applications

For as long as they have been in practical business use, computers have been used to file data, reassemble information into new formats, and perform logical operations and calculations. An exciting trend evident in computer problem solving is in the growth in the applicability of expert systems. These rely on stored facts and rules

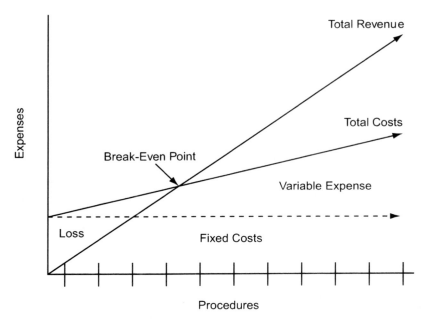

Figure 9–5   Break-Even Chart

of thumb to mimic the decision making of human experts. This has been success-ful when applied to narrowly defined tasks, but we still lack a system that pos-sesses common sense.

YOUR INTUITIVE PROCESS: KEY TO CREATIVE PROBLEM SOLVING

Give your intuitive process time to act. Set aside some think time each day. Cap-ture thoughts as they occur, like the ringing of a muted telephone. These are most likely to pop up when your logical thought process is on hold. Turn off conscious cerebration to let your cerebral energy flow into your unconscious mind. Day-dreaming, relaxation, and meditation help. Walking, jogging, and other kinds of exercise increase cerebral blood flow, and this improves the thought generation process. Solitude can be effective, particularly when it is enhanced by listening to ocean sounds (real or recorded) or background music.

Pay attention to the nagging doubts you feel when you are trying to make a deci-sion. They may represent experience stored in your unconscious mind. A strategy

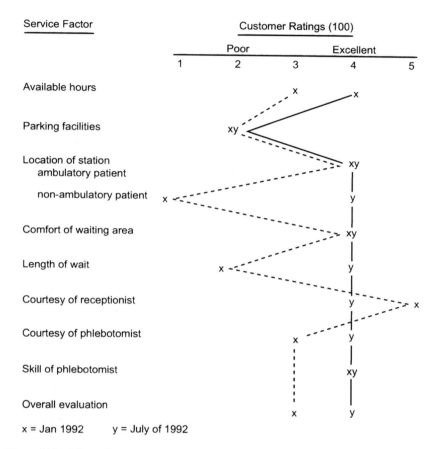

Figure 9–6 Likert Chart

espoused by Dr. Joyce Brothers, the well-known television psychologist, is to think about a problem just before dropping off to sleep.[4]

Simple Way to Stimulate Your Intuitive Process

Document your problem at the top of a sheet of paper. Under this heading, number the lines 1 through 20. Now force yourself to write down 20 solutions. The first few will come easily (these are usually the ones that you have already considered and discarded). Subsequent alternatives surface with increasing difficulty and are more likely to have originated in your unconscious mind and are more inspirational.[5]

GROUP PROBLEM SOLVING

A problem of any appreciable scope is like a world globe. From any one spot you cannot see all of the globe. Neither does any one person have an all-encompassing view. In group problem solving, more ideas are generated. An added bonus is that a group is more likely to support the choice it made.

Group discussions increase the likelihood of serendipity, the fortuitous result of two or more elements or events accidentally coming together to create an opportunity. When people put their heads together, they come up with more solutions than when they work individually. With this synergy, one plus one can readily equal three.

Importance of Consensus

A group often makes decisions before all the opinions of the members have been explored. Participants who are not heard from may leave a meeting angry. They may not support the implementation of the decisions. A few will even sabotage the initiative. A consensus prevents such occurrences (Exhibit 9–1).

A consensus is a genuine meeting of the minds. It is not reached by voting. Even a unanimous vote does not represent a consensus if some members are denied an opportunity to speak up. With a consensus some members may prefer different solutions, but after full and fair discussion they agree that they can live with what the group decided. Be wary of the possibility of the Abilene Paradox.

CREATIVE PROBLEM-SOLVING GROUPS

Unstructured Brainstorming Groups

Unstructured meetings are little more than beer-and-pretzel gabfests, typically lots of talk, lots of wandering off the topic, and not much action. All too many com-

Exhibit 9–1 Basics of Consensus Decision Making

- Ensure that each person expresses his or her viewpoint fully.
- Avoid hasty conclusions or agreements.
- Explore the positive features of each alternative.
- Expose and analyze the negative features of each alternative.
- Resolve disagreements.
- Avoid techniques of voting, averaging, or bargaining.
- Insist that each member agree that he or she can live with the solution. If any member balks, you do not have a consensus.

mittee meetings degenerate into these kinds of sessions. There are exceptions, of course, especially when entrepreneurs or creative people get together.

Structured Brainstorming Groups

Structured brainstorming groups generate ideas guided by certain rules. Following is one technique:

1. A problem is presented to the group.
2. Each member thinks about the problem and records his or her ideas on a sheet of paper. No comment or discussion is allowed at this time.
3. Each member reads one item from his or her list. Each of these is recorded on a flip chart. No comment or discussion is permitted at this time either, but members may piggyback on the ideas of others.
4. This sequence is repeated until all the ideas are displayed on the chart.
5. Each item is then discussed, amplified, or modified. The originator of each item may be asked to leave the room while his or her idea is discussed. Criticism is now encouraged.
6. Each member ranks the items, and the votes are recorded on the chart.[6]

Note that there are two phases in this approach: the generation phase (Steps 1 through 4) and the evaluation phase (Steps 5 and 6).

To get the maximum benefit of brainstorming, make certain that participants know beforehand what is going to be discussed and encourage them to come loaded with ideas. Set a good example by bringing a large packet of your own suggestions, including some really wild ones. Even consider leading off with your wildest idea. And when brainstorming, never reject an idea out of hand because it sounds ridiculous, highly impractical, or downright stupid; you never know when a dumb idea will lead someone's thought processes to a workable solution.

Think About It

In making any but the simplest of decisions or addressing any but the most elementary of problems, it is always necessary to accept some risk and uncertainty, uncertainty in that you cannot be completely sure that the decision is absolutely the correct one and risk in that there are consequences to making the wrong decision. It is risk and uncertainty that make decision makers uneasy with the process, but if risk and uncertainty were both reduced to zero, there would be no need to decide because the answer would be self-evident.

Questions for Review and Discussion

1. What is the true difference between consultative leadership and participative leadership in decision making?

2. The chapter suggests how autocratic, consultative, and participative managers make decisions. How are bureaucratic managers likely to make decisions?
3. No matter how simple a decision situation seems to be, why can it be said that there are always at least two alternative choices available?
4. Isn't it the responsibility of the boss to make decisions and solve problems? Why push these activities down to employee level?
5. What is the primary drawback likely to be encountered in making a decision when the problem is not your problem?
6. In creative idea-generating situations, why should wild or foolish or even downright stupid-sounding ideas not be rejected as soon as they arise?
7. In diagnosing a problem, it is always necessary to be on guard against mistakenly labeling a problem symptom as the problem itself. What is most likely to happen if what is addressed is a problem symptom and not the causal problem?
8. Why might we say that ignoring or even forgetting a problem can itself be considered a decision?
9. What should be the ultimate determinant of how much time and effort is put into any particular decision situation?
10. What are the essential differences between decision by vote and decision by true consensus?

Case: More Pleasant Dreams

Imagine yourself as night-shift charge nurse on a medical-surgical unit. For several months you have had a problem with a staff nurse whose performance you consider unsatisfactory. She seems to continually take advantage of quiet times during her shift to doze off at the nursing station. You have reprimanded her several times for sleeping on the job, and you have reached the point where you believe you can no longer simply scold her for her conduct. Her position, however, is that "it's no big deal," that she's always certain to hear any call signals as long as she's at the nursing station. (Your hospital has a clear policy concerning written warnings, but policy is relatively loose concerning oral warnings; these can be unlimited and issued at your discretion, so you can deliver as many as you believe necessary.)

For a written warning to become official and entered into an employee's personnel file, it must be agreed to and countersigned by the unit's nurse manager and the director of nursing. You issued the offending nurse two written warnings; both warnings cleared through the unit manager. However, you believe you can go no further without backing from the office of the director of nursing, and there has been no follow-up from that direction. Meanwhile, the employee continues to be a problem.

Questions

1. What would your decision be concerning the sleeping employee if it were not necessary to clear such actions through the director of nursing?
2. Assuming you have indeed "hit a wall" as described in the final paragraph of the case, what would you consider doing to try to get some action or support?
3. If you feel stuck with the reality of having your personnel decisions approved—or essentially made—by higher management, what information would you assemble and how would you prepare yourself to try getting a decision favorable to you from your chain of command?
4. What is the director of nursing actually doing by reserving the right to approve or veto your decisions?

Case: The Long-Time Employee

Assume you have been head nurse of the same medical-surgical unit for nearly 20 years. One of your employees, a licensed practical nurse named Hilda, has been part of the unit's day shift for even longer than you have been head nurse. In fact, Hilda is the only original member remaining of the crew that existed when you first took over the unit.

About 6 months ago Hilda returned to work after an extensive illness that left her noticeably changed in a number of ways. Where once she was energetic and seemed to possess considerable stamina, now the hustle and bustle of the day shift and always being on her feet and on the move seem to wear her down rapidly. You have felt a growing concern for Hilda, and for the rest of the team as well, because it has become obvious to you that Hilda is not bearing her share of the load. Other members of your already overworked crew are working extra hard to make up the difference.

Your concern reached a peak this week when three of your staff nurses came to talk to you about Hilda. Although they came with apparent reluctance—Hilda had always been well liked by both staff and patients—they were quite convinced that something had to be done for both Hilda's sake and the sake of the department. It seems that Hilda has barely been able to accomplish half of what she should be expected to do in an 8-hour shift.

Hilda knows only nursing; she has been an LPN for all of her working life. She will not be eligible for retirement for 5 more years.

It is evident that you need to make a decision concerning Hilda and her apparent inability to keep up with the work. Identify at least three alternatives (or more, if you wish) that you believe might be possible solutions.

Questions

1. Which alternative appears sufficiently workable to be the first one attempted? And what information do you need to assemble in preparing to justify your decision?
2. If your initial decision is found unworkable or unacceptable, which alternative would be your second choice? Why?

REFERENCES

1. Lewin, K. 1951. *Field theory in social science*. New York: Harper & Row.
2. Gantt, H. 1973. *Industrial leadership*. Easton, PA: Hive.
3. Likert, R. 1961. *New patterns of management*. New York: McGraw-Hill.
4. Sullivan, D. 1987. *Work smart, not hard*. New York: Facts on File.
5. DeBono, E. 1970. *Lateral thinking: Creativity step by step*. New York: Harper & Row.
6. Delbecq, A. L., et al. 1975. *Group techniques for program planning*. Glenview, IL: Scott-Foresman.

INDEX

CPSIA information can be obtained at www.ICGtesting.com
Printed in the USA
LVOW132005070413

327975LV00002B/51/P

9 781449 629236